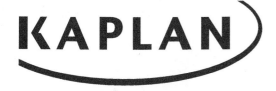

6 Practice Tests for the

BMAT

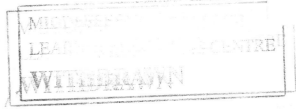
Second Edition

D1614630

BMAT is a registered trademark of Cambridge ... r sponsors nor endorses this product.

Special thanks to the team who made this book possible:

Simone Abbou, Mia Akanni, Laura Barnard, Alessandra Booth, Kim Bowers, Matthew Callan, Louise Cook, Scarlet Edmonds, Joanna Graham, Brian Holmes, Martin Kalushkov, Taha Khan, Corinne Morgan, Asha Przybyl, Teresa Rupp, Nimesh Shah

BMAT is a registered trademark of Cambridge Assessment, which neither sponsors nor endorses this product.

This publication is designed to provide accurate information in regard to the subject matter covered as of its publication date, with the understanding that knowledge and best practice constantly evolve. The publisher is not engaged in rendering medical, legal, accounting, or other professional service. If medical or legal advice or other expert assistance is required, the services of a competent professional should be sought. This publication is not intended for use in clinical practice or the delivery of medical care. To the fullest extent of the law, neither the Publisher nor the Editors assume any liability for any injury and/or damage to persons or property arising out of or related to any use of the material contained in this book.

TABLE OF CONTENTS

TEST 1

Test 1 Answer Grids 3

Test 1 7

TEST 2

Test 2 Answer Grids 51

Test 2 55

TEST 3

Test 3 Answer Grids 97

Test 3 101

TEST 4

Test 4 Answer Grids 145

Test 4 149

TEST 5

Test 5 Answer Grids 193

Test 5 197

TEST 6

Test 6 Answer Grids 241

Test 6 245

HOW TO USE THIS BOOK

If You Bought This Book By Itself...

You're serious about going to medical school. You wouldn't have opened this book otherwise. This book can help you to achieve your goal. It will give you realistic practice on the BMAT, so you are ready to do your best on Test Day.

There are two main components to your BMAT practice package: this book and your Online Centre.

- This book contains six full-length BMAT practice tests, each with answer sheets, answer keys and scoring tables.
- Your Online Centre includes explanations for each test, printable answer sheets and test updates.

Getting Started

1. Register your Online Centre.
2. Take a BMAT Diagnostic Test to identify your strengths and weaknesses.
3. Create a study plan.
4. Use the remaining tests to improve your pacing and performance.

Step 1: Register Your Online Centre

Use these simple steps to register your Online Centre:

1. Go to **kaptest.com/moreonline**.
2. Follow the onscreen instructions. Please have a copy of your book available.

Access to the Online Centre is limited to the original owner of this book and is nontransferable. Kaplan is not responsible for providing access to the Online Centre to customers who purchase or borrow used copies of this book. Access to the Online Centre for this edition expires one year from the date of registration.

Step 2: Take a BMAT Practice Test

It's a good idea to take a practice test early on. Doing so will give you the initial feedback and diagnostic information you need to achieve your maximum score.

Use Test 1 in this book as your diagnostic test. It will give you a chance to familiarise yourself with the various sections and question types. It will also allow you to accurately gauge the pacing required for each section, so you can identify the sections where you will need to practise for pacing as well as accuracy.

We recommend that you print out answer sheets from the Online Centre and use these as you complete the test. Be sure to sit the test under timed conditions. Then, check your answers against the answer key at the end of the test and use the scoring tables to determine your scaled scores. Make a note of these scores, as they will serve as a baseline for your performance on subsequent practice tests.

Review the explanations for every question in the Online Centre to better understand your performance. Look for patterns in the questions you answered correctly and incorrectly. Were you stronger in some areas than others? This analysis will help you target your practice to specific concepts.

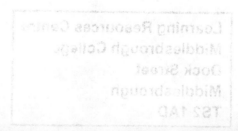

Step 3: Create a Study Plan

Use what you've learned from your diagnostic test to identify areas for closer study and practice. Think about how many hours you can consistently devote to BMAT study. Be sure to practise for accuracy – answering questions correctly – as well as for pacing – answering questions quickly. Most students find they must improve accuracy before they work on pacing.

Schedule time for study, practice and review. Find blocks of time where you can fit in revision and practice. Don't overlook any opportunities for short bursts of intense revision. You will gain more if you revise for an hour a day than if you try to revise all day on a Saturday or Sunday. Use weekends (or days when you have more time) to sit and review practice tests. Check in with yourself frequently to make sure you're not falling behind your plan or forgetting about any of your resources.

Step 4: Use the Remaining Tests to Improve Your Pacing and Performance

Be sure to sit each BMAT practice test under timed conditions. Make any notes or rough working in this book, just as you would write on the test booklet on Test Day. You may find that you need to practise specific skills for some sections of the exam, such as doing maths without a calculator or planning your points before writing the essay.

One of the most common errors in approaching BMAT revision is to sit practice tests and not review them thoroughly. Review time is your best chance to increase your score. Full-length practice tests will also help you build up your endurance – pacing yourself within each section and also across the entire exam, so you are ready to maintain your energy and accuracy for two hours and maximise your marks in all three BMAT sections.

Thanks for choosing Kaplan. We wish you the best of luck on your journey to BMAT success.

If You Bought the BMAT Complete Self-Study Programme...

First, follow the instructions on the sheet of paper that came with your book to register to receive your Online Study Plan. Your online materials include 10 hours of video lessons, the *BMAT Strategy* ebook, 800+ practice questions in the BMAT Question Bank, as well as overall guidance for how to use all of your study resources.

Note that you will have two choices for how to complete each BMAT practice test:

1. Take the test online.
2. Take the test in this book.

Option 1: Take the test online

Your Online Study Plan includes three links for each practice test: Section 1, Section 2 and Section 3.

For Section 1 and Section 2, the online testing interface will time you as you work through the questions. You must launch each section separately from the webpage. Do any rough working or notations on scrap paper as you complete the test.

You will receive your scores for Section 1 and Section 2 upon completing the test. You can then review the explanations for all questions from Section 1 and Section 2 in the testing interface.

For Section 3, follow the instructions online for how to complete your essay and submit it for grading if you wish.

Option 2: Take the test in this book

Time yourself as you sit the test using this book. Before you begin, you may prefer to download the answer sheets from your Online Study Plan and print them out. Note that there are different answer sheets for each Section 1 and Section 2; the answer sheet is the same for all versions of Section 3. Do any rough working or notations in this book as you complete the test.

Check your answers against the answer key at the end of the test and use the scoring tables to determine your scaled scores. Make a note of these scores, so you can track your progress as you work through the remaining practice tests.

Review the explanations for Section 1 and Section 2 in the explanation booklets (PDF) in your Online Study Plan.

For Section 3, follow the online instructions to submit your essay for each practice test.

Thanks for choosing Kaplan. We wish you the best of luck on your journey to BMAT success.

Test 1

BMAT
Section 1

Test ID

Test 1 ●   Test 2 ○   Test 3 ○

Last Name

First Name

Date

Completely fill in the space for your intended answer choice

A B C D E
○ ○ ● ○ ○

1   A B C D E F G H   ○ ○ ○ ○ ○ ○ ○ ○

2   A B C D E F   ○ ○ ○ ○ ○ ○

3   A B C D E   ○ ○ ○ ○ ○

4   A B C D E F G   ○ ○ ○ ○ ○ ○ ○

5   A B C D   ○ ○ ○ ○

6   A B C D   ○ ○ ○ ○

7   A B C D E   ○ ○ ○ ○ ○

8   A B C D E   ○ ○ ○ ○ ○

9   A B C D E F   ○ ○ ○ ○ ○ ○

10   A B C D E   ○ ○ ○ ○ ○

11   A B C D   ○ ○ ○ ○

12   A B C D E F G H   ○ ○ ○ ○ ○ ○ ○ ○

13   A B C D E   ○ ○ ○ ○ ○

14   A B C D E   ○ ○ ○ ○ ○

15   A B C D   ○ ○ ○ ○

16   A B C D E F   ○ ○ ○ ○ ○ ○

17   A B C D   ○ ○ ○ ○

18   A B C D   ○ ○ ○ ○

19   A B C D   ○ ○ ○ ○

20   A B C D   ○ ○ ○ ○

21   A B C D E F   ○ ○ ○ ○ ○ ○

22   A B C D E   ○ ○ ○ ○ ○

23   A B C D   ○ ○ ○ ○

24   A B C D   ○ ○ ○ ○

25   A B C D   ○ ○ ○ ○

26   A B C D E   ○ ○ ○ ○ ○

27   A B C D E   ○ ○ ○ ○ ○

28   A B C D E   ○ ○ ○ ○ ○

29   A B C D E   ○ ○ ○ ○ ○

30   A B C D E F   ○ ○ ○ ○ ○ ○

31   A B C D E   ○ ○ ○ ○ ○

32   A B C D   ○ ○ ○ ○

33   A B C D E F G H   ○ ○ ○ ○ ○ ○ ○ ○

34   A B C D   ○ ○ ○ ○

35   A B C D   ○ ○ ○ ○

BMAT is a registered trademark of Cambridge Assessment, which neither sponsors nor endorses this product.

K   3

BMAT
Section 2

KAPLAN
TEST PREP

Test ID Test 1 ● Test 2 ○ Test 3 ○

Last Name

First Name

Date

Completely fill in the space for your intended answer choice

A B C D E
○ ○ ● ○ ○

1 A B C D E
   ○ ○ ○ ○ ○

2 A B C D E
   ○ ○ ○ ○ ○

3 A B C D E
   ○ ○ ○ ○ ○

4 A B C D
   ○ ○ ○ ○

5 A B C D
   ○ ○ ○ ○

6 A B C D
   ○ ○ ○ ○

7 A B C D
   ○ ○ ○ ○

8 A B C D E
   ○ ○ ○ ○ ○

9 A B C D E
   ○ ○ ○ ○ ○

10 A B C D E
    ○ ○ ○ ○ ○

11 A B C D
    ○ ○ ○ ○

12 A B C D E
    ○ ○ ○ ○ ○

13 A B C D
    ○ ○ ○ ○

14 A B C D
    ○ ○ ○ ○

15 A B C D
    ○ ○ ○ ○

16 A B C D E F G
    ○ ○ ○ ○ ○ ○ ○

17 A B C D
    ○ ○ ○ ○

18 A B C D E
    ○ ○ ○ ○ ○

19 A B C D
    ○ ○ ○ ○

20 A B C D E
    ○ ○ ○ ○ ○

21 A B C D
    ○ ○ ○ ○

22 A B C D E
    ○ ○ ○ ○ ○

23 A B C D
    ○ ○ ○ ○

24 A B C D
    ○ ○ ○ ○

25 A B C D E
    ○ ○ ○ ○ ○

26 A B C D
    ○ ○ ○ ○

27 A B C D E
    ○ ○ ○ ○ ○

BMAT
Section 3

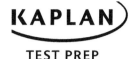

	Test 1	Test 2	Test 3	Test 4	Test 5	Test 6
Test ID	○	○	○	○	○	○

Last Name

First Name

Question answered ☐

Your answer must be contained within this area.

BMAT is a registered trademark of Cambridge Assessment, which neither sponsors nor endorses this product.

5

BMAT SECTION 1: APTITUDE AND SKILLS (60 MINUTES)

You have 60 minutes to answer 35 questions. There are no penalties for incorrect answers, so you should attempt all questions.

Fill in your answers to each question on the answer sheet provided. Shade the circles corresponding to the answer choice(s) you have selected.

Avoid making stray marks on the paper. If you make a mistake, erase your answer completely and try again.

Calculators are **not** permitted.

1 A patient with diabetes is asked to record her blood sugar readings when fasting and two hours after eating over ten days, both in mmol/L.

Day	Fasting	Two hours after eating	Hb1Ac
Wed am	4.7	6.1	6.2%
Wed pm	6.1	8.6	5.8%
Thu am	4.5	6.4	7.0%
Thu pm	5.9	7.1	6.5%
Fri am	7.2	9.7	4.3%
Fri pm	5.9	9.4	5.7%
Sat am	5.4	8.3	4.4%
Sat pm	5.2	6.9	5.9%
Sun am	6.8	9.2	6.3%
Sun pm	5.5	6.8	5.4%
Mon am	4.8	9.1	6.8%
Mon pm	6.4	9.3	4.1%
Tue am	5.7	8.4	5.2%
Tue pm	6.6	7.8	5.7%
Wed am	6.2	10.3	7.1%
Wed pm	4.6	8.2	4.9%
Thu am	5.3	8.0	4.4%
Thu pm	3.9	8.1	6.3%
Fri am	5.5	9.7	6.2%
Fri pm	7.1	8.9	7.3%

The patient also records her HbA1c levels two hours after eating. A person with diabetes is recommended to have an HbA1c level less than 7.0%, whilst someone without diabetes would normally be less than 5.7%.

What was the patient's HbA1c level when she had the biggest difference between blood sugar levels when fasting and two hours after eating?

A 4.3%

B 4.4%

C 4.9%

D 5.7%

E 6.2%

F 6.3%

G 6.8%

H 7.1%

2   Rachel painted a room 70% green and 30% eggshell.

Before she started, she had three full 2.5 litre pots of paint: one yellow, one blue and one white. She mixed equal parts yellow and blue to create the green paint and she mixed yellow and white in the ratio 1 : 5 to create the eggshell paint.

She mixed the exact amounts of green and eggshell paint that she needed. After mixing the paints, Rachel had 750 ml of blue paint left.

How much of the yellow paint did Rachel have left?

A   250 ml

B   300 ml

C   375 ml

D   450 ml

E   500 ml

F   600 ml

3   A recent study of unmarried rugby players concluded that unmarried players had considerably longer professional careers than did married players. Therefore, rugby players who aspire to long, professional careers should not get married.

Which one of the following is the best statement of the flaw in the above argument?

A   It assumes that all rugby players wish to play professionally.

B   It ignores the fact that some athletes have more natural ability than others.

C   It assumes that the length of a player's professional career is caused by marital status.

D   It ignores that marriage can provide rugby players with many emotional and financial benefits.

E   It assumes that spouses of rugby players object to long, professional careers.

4   My internet banking passcode consists of six digits. None of the digits are repeated.

The fifth digit is 4.

If you break the passcode into three 2-digit numbers, these three numbers add up to 130.

If you break the passcode into two 3-digit numbers, these two numbers add up to 400.

What is the last digit of my passcode?

A   1

B   2

C   3

D   5

E   6

F   7

G   8

5   When the clock in a school's clock tower breaks, students decide to hang a series of paddles on a wall to show the time from 12:00 AM to 11:59 PM. Each paddle contains one digit or the AM or PM mark. In the diagram below, the time is shown as 9:35 PM.

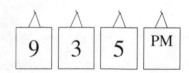

How many paddles are necessary for the clock to function properly?

A   27

B   28

C   29

D   34

6   A recent study tracked two groups of children for twenty-four months from birth: one group that was taught infant sign language from birth and a control group that did not learn to sign. At twelve months, the non-signing children had an average vocabulary of two to three words. At eighteen months, the non-signing children knew between ten and fifty words; some of these children were able to form simple sentences. Meanwhile, the children who were taught to sign knew an average of twenty-five signs and sixteen spoken words at twelve months, and most could string together signs and words into simple sentences. This goes to show that …

Which of the following most logically completes the last sentence in the above passage?

A   … babies will learn words if they are encouraged to communicate with their parents.

B   … teaching newborn babies to sign will increase their linguistic development.

C   … babies that learn to sign will start speaking at an earlier age than babies that do not learn to sign.

D   … newborn babies that learn to sign will be less comfortable speaking than signing.

7   Spiffy Cleaning Service's fees are based on a base fee for a scheduled appointment and an additional fee per room cleaned.

It costs Nigel £17 to have his four-room flat cleaned, and it would cost Priscilla, Nigel's neighbour across the hall, £14 to have her three-room flat cleaned.

If the cleaning service agreed to schedule Nigel and Priscilla for one, joint appointment to clean seven rooms, how much would it cost?

A   £22

B   £23

C   £25

D   £26

E   £29

Questions 8 to 11 refer to the following information:

The pie charts below show the various reasons for people being admitted to Accident & Emergency in the United States and Great Britain over a 12 month period to the nearest 5%. The total annual admittance rates are 2,000 per 10,000 people in the United States and 1,500 per 10,000 people in Great Britain. The population of the United States is assumed to be five times larger than the population of Great Britain.

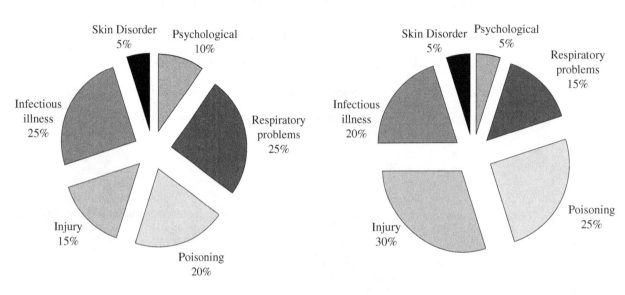

8   For both Americans and Britons, approximately how many individuals per 10,000 per year were admitted for skin disorders?

   A   75

   B   87

   C   95

   D   100

   E   110

9   For which problem was the number of admittances per 1,000 higher in Great Britain than in the United States?

   A   Respiratory

   B   Poisoning

   C   Injury

   D   Infectious Illness

   E   Skin Disorder

   F   Psychological

10   Which of the columns below shows the number of admittances of Americans per 10,000 per year for each disease?

	A	B	C	D	E
Respiratory problems	225	375	300	550	500
Poisoning	375	300	500	475	400
Injury	450	225	600	325	300
Infectious illness	300	375	400	550	500
Skin disorder	75	75	100	150	100
Psychological problems	75	150	100	325	200

11   In which of the following bar charts is the proportion of admittance by ailment in the UK correctly shown?

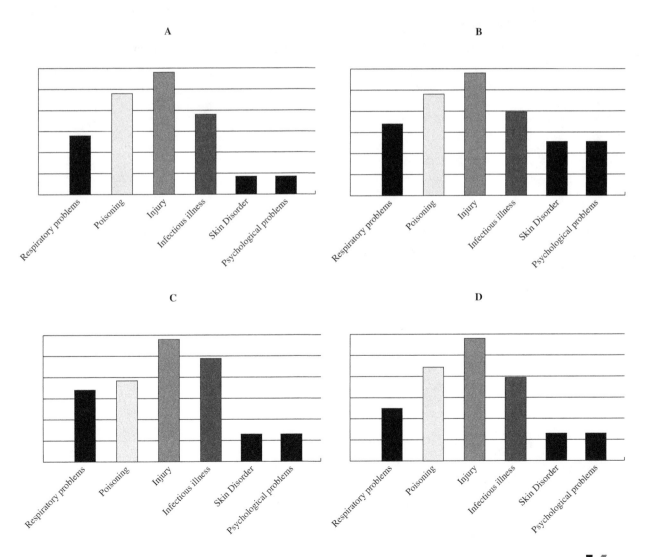

A

B

C

D

12   The graph below shows the how the heart rate of a person exercising varies with time.

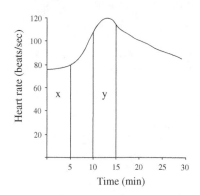

The area marked y on the graph is 1.5 times as large as the area marked x on the graph.

Which of the following statements must be true?

1   The average heart rate is one-and-a-half times as great between 10 and 15 minutes as it is between naught and five minutes.

2   The heart rate increases one-and-a-half times as rapidly between 10 and 15 minutes as it does between 0 and 5 minutes.

3   The heart rate after 15 minutes is one-and-a-half times what it is after 5 minutes.

4   The number of heart beats between 10 and 15 minutes is one-and-a-half times the number of beats between 0 and 5 minutes.

A   1 only

B   1 and 2

C   1 and 3

D   1 and 4

E   1, 2 and 3

F   1, 2 and 4

G   2, 3 and 4

H   all of them

13   The graph below shows the number of kilometres people of various ages tend to live from their places of employment.

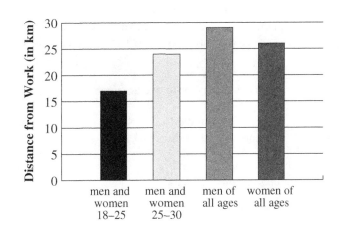

Which of the following information can be deduced from the information provided?

    1   Men are likely to live further from work as they age.

    2   Men and women tend to live further from work than in the past.

    3   24-year-old adults are likely to live closer to work than 50-year-old adults.

A   1 and 2

B   2 and 3

C   1 and 3

D   1, 2 and 3

E   none of them

14   A Member of Parliament is trying to introduce a measure for debate that would outlaw the use of mobile phones in restaurants across the UK. His office has fielded calls from his constituency that were overwhelmingly in favour of the proposed law. Restaurant owners are lining up to support the ban on mobile phones, claiming that their patrons are fed up with inconsiderate mobile phone use in restaurants. Parliament should not defer to mobile phone service providers on this issue because the measure would still allow patrons to use their phones within a one-meter radius of public phones inside of a restaurant.

Which one of the following is an underlying assumption of the above argument?

A   Mobile phone companies will protest this measure.

B   The Member of Parliament's constituency is representative of the UK as a whole.

C   Enforcement of this ban would fall on the shoulders of restaurant owners.

D   Most mobile phone users inside restaurants make an effort to talk quietly.

E   The callers to the Member of Parliament's office were actually from his district.

15   A minimum drinking age of 21 should be established in the UK. Half of all crimes committed by people under the age of 21 are perpetrated while the suspect is under the influence of alcohol. Most youth surveyed said they would most likely do better in school if a minimum drinking age of 21 were instituted and strictly enforced. Raising the minimum drinking age to 21 would keep unruly youngsters from the mayhem and anarchy of drunken rages. Also, the risk of cirrhosis of the liver tends to be increased when subjects begin drinking at ages under 21.

Which of the following, if true, most weakens the above argument?

A   With a minimum drinking age of 21 in the United States, the rate of crime among youth where alcohol is involved is the same as in the UK.

B   The study of liver damage versus drinking age did not take into account that those who drank early also tended to have parents with liver disease.

C   The statistics for the crime rate are from England only.

D   Recent studies indicate that equivalent amounts of alcohol have less effect on the reflexes of people under the age of 25 than older individuals.

16   The Atlantic Cinema screened all three *Godfather* films in order three times, starting one evening and ending the following day.

The running times of the films were as follows:

The Godfather	-	177 minutes
The Godfather Part II	-	200 minutes
The Godfather Part III	-	162 minutes

The film times were arranged so that the first screening of the first film started at 18:00 the first day and the third screening of the final film finished at 23:45 the following day. The interval between successive films was the same throughout both days.

How long was each interval between successive films?

A   11 minutes

B   12 minutes

C   15 minutes

D   16 minutes

E   21 minutes

F   24 minutes

17 Six friends, William, Camilla, Liam, Andrew, Rose and Harriet, all want to play pinball at an arcade for the second time in 2 weeks. They must decide the order in which they will play. They have decided that no one will follow the same person in order of play that they followed the previous week. Also, Liam insists that all of the women (Harriet, Rose and Camilla) go before him.

The order in which they played the previous week is as follows:

Liam, Harriet, William, Andrew, Rose and Camilla

Which **one** of the following orders **may** be correct?

A   Rose, Harriet, Camilla, William, Andrew, Liam

B   Harriet, Rose, Camilla, Liam, Andrew, William

C   Andrew, Harriet, Camilla, Liam, William, Rose

D   Camilla, Rose, Andrew, Harriet, Liam, William

Questions 18 to 21 refer to the following information:

A landlord owns two different blocks of flats in the same neighbourhood, the Regal Court and Covenant Mansion. The Regal Court was renovated two years ago and the rents, on average, are higher than at Covenant Mansion. The tenants in flats 3B, 2C and 1A of Covenant Mansion have recently moved out and the landlord must decide if he wants to renovate the three flats in order to raise the rent. If he does, he can charge 1.5 times what each flat rents for currently.

The tenants' rents and the size of their respective flats is shown in the table below (before the three tenants moved out).

Regal Court			Covenant Mansion		
Flat No.	Size (in m^2)	Rent (£)	Flat No.	Size (in m^2)	Rent (£)
1A	75	800	1A	85	600
1B	80	900	1B	100	750
1C	90	1,100	1C	60	425
1D	100	1,150	2A	85	650
2A	70	775	2B	100	675
2B	80	850	2C	65	450
2C	90	1,000	3A	85	625
2D	100	1,200	3B	100	700
			3C	65	475

18   What is the average rent at Covenant Mansion just after the three tenants move out?

A   £450

B   £594

C   £600

D   £996

19   By how much will the total rent for Covenant Mansion rise (from its previous full occupancy amount) if the renovations are completed?

A   £875

B   £900

C   £1,225

D   £1,400

20   If the landlord renovates and then all of the rents rise by 5% in a year (except the newly renovated flats, which stay at their new level), what will the total income from rent be for one month for both buildings?

    A   £11,943.75

    B   £14,068.75

    C   £14,568.75

    D   £14,700.00

21   The following chart shows a best fit line for the current rents plotted against the size of each flat. Which flat is furthest below the best fit line?

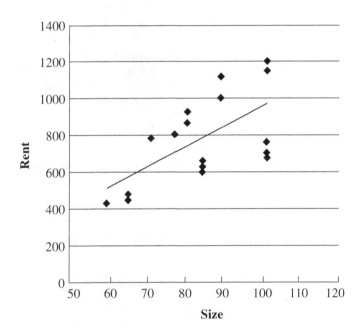

    A   The Regal Court 1A

    B   The Regal Court 1D

    C   The Regal Court 2A

    D   Covenant Mansion 2A

    E   Covenant Mansion 2B

    F   Covenant Mansion 3A

22 Every year, the effectiveness of antibiotics in fighting infection is lowered as more and more bacteria develop a resistance to those antibiotics that are most commonly used. If this trend continues, the world will eventually see a global health crisis as doctors lose their ability to adequately fight infection in patients. Doctors must be educated about this looming medical emergency and instructed that the only way to slow this process is to write fewer prescriptions for antibiotics which are not necessary.

Which **one** of the following is an underlying assumption of the above argument?

A Not enough new antibiotics will be developed in the coming years to counter the trend.

B Doctors are not concerned about the implications of writing prescriptions for antibiotics so freely.

C Some antibiotics have become ineffective in preventing infection.

D Doctors will write fewer prescriptions if instructed to do so.

E The prescribing of antibiotics can be lessened without undue risk to the general public.

23 A large-scale clinical trial in Britain has shown, at a very high level of statistical significance, that those who live in large cities and do not own an automobile are four times less likely to suffer from high blood pressure than those who own at least one car and live in a large city. Researchers have concluded that the stress of owning and operating a car in a large city is a significant health risk.

Which **one** of the following is a reason why this conclusion might be unsafe?

A Those who do not own an automobile walk an average of 1.5km per day more than those who own a vehicle.

B Comparable studies in Germany have been largely inconclusive.

C There is not enough data to suggest that the life expectancy of automobile owners is less than that of non-owners.

D A series of surveys found that the most stressful part of driving in large cities is the danger of hitting a pedestrian.

24 Over a period of time, 1 200 people in a small town contract influenza. 60% are children under 18 years of age, and 55% of the adults (18 or older) who contract the virus are 65 years of age or older. On average, 5 in 20 people who contract the virus visit a doctor for treatment.

Assuming that all sufferers are equally likely to visit a doctor for treatment, what is the most likely number of adults under 65 who visit a doctor for treatment?

A 27

B 54

C 216

D 270

25 The price of a piece of merchandise is marked up 60%. The price is later reduced by 50% on clearance. By what percentage would the price have to be increased to reach its original level?

    A   25%

    B   40%

    C   80%

    D   125%

26 Many people think a vegan diet – one that does not include any animal products, such as eggs or milk – must be less healthy than a diet that includes meat, eggs and dairy. Yet extensive medical research has shown that the opposite is the case. On average, vegan adults are 10 to 20 pounds lighter than meat-eating adults, who have a higher incidence of weight-related issues, such as diabetes, heart problems and high blood pressure. Processed meats such as bacon and sausage have been proven to cause cancer, and saturated fats in meat can cause breast cancer and dementia. It's true that vegans must take care to ensure a steady supply of iron, calcium and vitamin D, but the risk of not eating a balanced diet is a potential problem for everyone, not just vegans.

Which one of the following best expresses the conclusion of the above argument?

    A   Vegans have a greater risk of not consuming enough nutrients.

    B   People are not aware of the health risks of a vegan diet.

    C   A vegan diet is healthier than a meat-based diet.

    D   Eating a vegan diet ensures you will weigh less and lower your risk of health problems.

    E   Processed meats and saturated fats are the worst foods to eat in terms of potential health risks.

27   In the past 5 years deforestation has claimed 10 000 km^2 of rainforest in South America. In response to this, many global environmental groups have pushed for bans on the "slash and burn" tactic of clearing land. But local farmers cannot be expected to abide by any such bans if they have no other option for gaining clear land for ranching and farming.

Which of the following are underlying assumptions of the above argument?

  1   Farmers have other options for gaining arable land to cultivate.

  2   Farmers participate in the deforestation.

  3   "Slash and burn" is the predominant method of clearing rainforest.

A   1 only

B   1 and 2 only

C   2 only

D   2 and 3 only

E   1, 2 and 3

28   Forensic dogs are three times as effective as the best X-ray machines at uncovering contraband such as drugs or explosives. Customs offices, whose primary function is to uncover concealed contraband, would save money by replacing their x-ray machines with teams of trained dogs.

The writer's failure to prove which one of the following renders the argument questionable?

A   Teams of trained dogs would be able to detect even new designer drugs.

B   Teams of trained dogs would be more cost effective than x-ray machines.

C   Teams of trained dogs do not get sick more often than x-ray machines break down.

D   X-ray machines do not serve some function other than uncovering contraband.

E   X-ray machines are cheaper to maintain than teams of trained dogs.

29 Five friends, Angus, Bernard, Cecil, Danielle and Elinor, have made reservations at a restaurant for dinner. Cecil arrives first and sits with his back to the wall. Danielle arrives next and sits to Cecil's right. Elinor arrives next and sits next to the window. Bernard sits next to Danielle. When Angus arrives, he asks to sit in Cecil's. Cecil agrees and takes one of the two remaining seats.

Which of the following could show how the five friends were sitting once they all arrived?

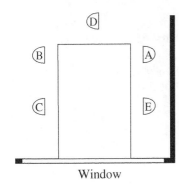
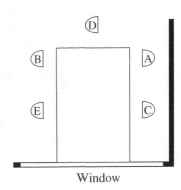
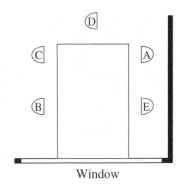

Window   Window   Window

A   1 only

B   2 only

C   3 only

D   1 and 2 only

E   2 and 3 only

30 There are three types of goals in the sport of Fishball:

- a head, which scores 7 points

- a fin, which scores 3 points

- a tail, which scores 2 points

The Dolphins scored a total of 840 points last season, setting a new record for each type of goal in the National Fishball League. In their record-breaking season, the Dolphins scored 58 heads and 91 tails.

Which one of the following pie charts indicates how many of the 840 points scored by the Dolphins last season were from heads, how many were from fins and how many were from tails?

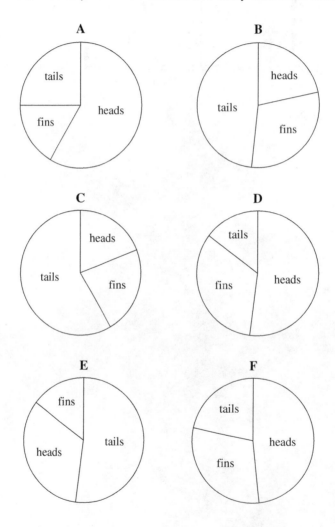

31 There are 150 slots in a cross-country bicycle race in which 7 teams are competing. After the time trials, each of the teams has placed no more than 30 cyclists in the race. No two teams have the same number of cyclists competing in the race.

What is the smallest number of cyclists that the fourth largest team can have?

A   14

B   15

C   16

D   17

E   18

Questions 32 to 35 refer to the following information:

It seems we can't go a week without a news story about the spending habits of millennials, generally defined as young adults aged 20 to 35. These stories are generally quite negative, trumpeting the latest expensive millennial habits, such as avocado toast and fancy coffees. There are a lot of millennials in the UK: 13.9% of the national population of 66,040,200 are millennials, with 19% of millennials living in London. Are these news stories fair to UK millennials, or are these young adults not the reckless spenders we have been led to expect?

A recent survey by Barclays suggests that many of these claims about millennials are overblown. Their research reveals that 70% of millennials in the UK set a monthly budget, the highest rate of any age group. Whilst there are surely some millennials that spend wildly without regard to financial planning, they are clearly a relatively small minority. Barclays found as well that 70% of millennials in the UK use their mobiles for banking and other financial purposes such as setting a budget. Millennials are the only age group in the UK in which a majority uses mobile technology in this way. Thanks to their budgeting habits, the average millennial in the UK saves £159.89 per month.

The Barclays survey determined how much the average millennial spends per month on 'luxuries' such as takeaways, meals in restaurants and 'daily treats' such as coffees and gym memberships. The average UK millennial spends £3,312.72 per year on these luxuries. The regions with the highest and lowest monthly averages are listed in the table below.

Luxuries	Region with highest average monthly spend		Region with lowest average monthly spend	
clothes, shoes and accessories	North East	£92.04	East of England	£45.23
coffees and snacks	North East	£75.83	Yorkshire and the Humber	£28.92
gym, sports and cinema	Scotland	£64.78	South West	£21.53
restaurant meals	London	£78.11	North East	£48.60
socialising	South West	£103.81	East Midlands	£48.91
takeaways	London	£57.48	Yorkshire and the Humber	£34.77

There are a few factors that could explain why millennials feel more financial pressure than older generations. Since they are younger and earlier in their careers, millennials will be on lower salaries than people in their 40s or older. Older generations are also far more likely to own their house or flat, as housing prices were much lower in the 1990s and before, when these older Britons would have been the age that millennials are today.

By comparison, the UK has 3,849,000 households led by a millennial, and 59.37% of these households rent their house or flat. With 14.15% of UK households led by a millennial, this is the only age group where a majority of households are rented rather than owned. With lower salaries and higher housing prices, it follows that it is much harder for millennials to buy property than it was for older generations.

32   If the same proportion of millennials nationwide and living in London set a monthly budget, how many millennials living in London set a monthly budget, to the nearest hundred?

    A   1,185,600

    B   1,229,700

    C   1,294,800

    D   1,337,900

33   Which of the following, if true, would strengthen the claim that UK millennials are unique in their use of mobiles for banking and other financial tasks?

    1   Most people aged 70 and over in the UK pay bills with cheques and visit a bank branch for banking transactions.

    2   Most teenagers in the UK use banking apps on mobiles and tablets for all their banking transactions.

    3   Most people aged 36 to 55 in the UK use laptops or desktop computers for banking, budgeting and completing tax forms.

    A   1 only

    B   2 only

    C   3 only

    D   1 and 2 only

    E   1 and 3 only

    F   2 and 3 only

    G   1, 2 and 3

    H   none

34   Which of the following statements can be inferred from the information in the table and the text?

    A   The average millennial living in London spends over £1,000 a year on meals in restaurants.

    B   The average millennial in the UK spends £306 per month on 'luxuries' as defined by Barclays.

    C   Of those in the UK who save regularly, the average millennial saves between £1,980 and £1,990 per year.

    D   On average, millennials in Yorkshire and the Humber spend less than £500 per year on takeaways.

35   Households led by a millennial that rent account for what percentage of all UK households?

    A   8.4%

    B   8.9%

    C   9.6%

    D   10.1%

BMAT SECTION 2: SCIENTIFIC KNOWLEDGE AND APPLICATIONS
(30 MINUTES)

You have 30 minutes to answer 27 questions. There are no penalties for incorrect answers, so you should attempt all questions.

Fill in your answers to each question on the answer sheet provided. Shade the circles corresponding to the answer choice(s) you have selected.

Avoid making stray marks on the paper. If you make a mistake, erase your answer completely and try again.

Calculators are **not** permitted.

1   Polydactyly (a condition in which an individual has too many fingers or toes) is inherited in an autosomal dominant manner. The dominant allele, D, codes for polydactyly, while the recessive allele, d, is healthy.

The diagram shows a family tree for the inheritance of polydactyly. Shaded individuals suffer from the condition.

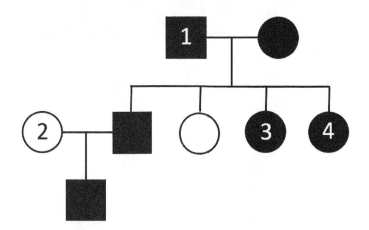

Individual 4 sees her doctor, who runs tests and tells her that, regardless of her partner, there is a 100% chance that her children will have polydactyly.

Which row of the table correctly identifies the genotypes of the four individuals labelled in the diagram?

	1	2	3	4
A	Dd	dd	DD or Dd	DD
B	DD or Dd	Dd	DD	DD
C	Dd	Dd	Dd	Dd
D	DD or Dd	dd	DD or Dd	DD or Dd
E	Dd	dd	DD or Dd	DD or Dd

2   Boron trifluoride can be prepared from a sodium tetraborate precursor according to the equation:

$$w\text{Na}_2\text{B}_4\text{O}_7 + x\text{CaF}_2 + y\text{SO}_3 \rightarrow z\text{BF}_3 + x\text{CaSO}_4 + w\text{Na}_2\text{SO}_4$$

What values of w, x, y and z are needed to balance this equation?

A $w = 2$ $x = 4$ $y = 12$ $z = 4$

B $w = 2$ $x = 12$ $y = 2$ $z = 8$

C $w = 1$ $x = 6$ $y = 4$ $z = 8$

D $w = 1$ $x = 6$ $y = 7$ $z = 4$

E $w = 1$ $x = 4$ $y = 5$ $z = 4$

3 Select the function that has the same y-intercept as $\dfrac{3y-5}{4} + \dfrac{17x}{2} = 5y + 3$.

A $\quad y = \dfrac{x}{2} - 1$

B $\quad y = 2x + 1$

C $\quad y = 17x + 3$

D $\quad y = 3x - 5$

E $\quad y = 5x + \dfrac{17}{2}$

4 The diagram below shows a section of a mechanical balance. What is the mass read to the correct number of significant figures?

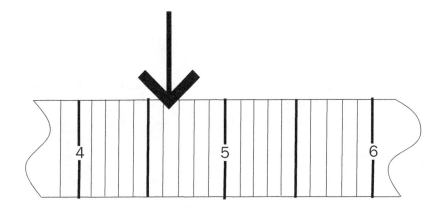

A	4.63 g		C	45 g
B	4.630 g		D	46.3 g

5   The graph below shows the oxygen saturation of hemoglobin at various partial pressures of oxygen (pO_2). The two different lines show the oxygen saturation curves at pH 7.4 and pH 7.2.

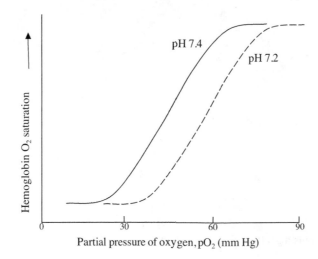

According to the graph, which of the following conditions would result in the greatest oxygen saturation?

A   pH 7.4, pO_2 60   **B**   pH 7.2, pO_2 70   **C**   pH 7.4, pO_2 40   **D**   pH 7.2, pO_2 50

6   A rectangular swimming pool 24 feet × 16 feet is filled to a height of 1 foot. How high would the same amount of water reach in a pool 20 feet × 8 feet?

A   0.42 feet

B   1.6 feet

C   2.4 feet

D   2.67 feet

7   A 100 watt motor uses how much electrical energy when connected to a 240 volt outlet for 30.0 minutes?

A   120 kJ

B   180 kJ

C   270 kJ

D   300 kJ

8   What is the correct path of food during digestion?

A   Oesophagus   →   Stomach   →   Small Intestine   →   Large Intestine

B   Oesophagus   →   Stomach   →   Large Intestine   →   Small Intestine

C   Trachea   →   Stomach   →   Small Intestine   →   Large Intestine

D   Trachea   →   Stomach   →   Large Intestine   →   Small Intestine

E   Oesophagus   →   Stomach   →   Small Intestine   →   Liver

9 Given that $32^y \times 2^z = 8^w$, express z in terms of w and y.

A $z = w - 3y$

B $z = 3w - 5y$

C $z = 5w - 3y$

D $z = 3w - y$

E $z = 0.6(wy)$

10 Which part of the neuron is mainly responsible for gathering input from neighbouring neurons or specialised receptors?

A	Axon	D	Dendrites
B	Pre-synaptic terminal	E	Nucleus
C	Cell body		

11 Which of the following is NOT a correct definition of the term *half-life?*

A   the time taken for the activity of a radioactive sample to halve

B   the time point halfway between the initial quantity of a radioactive sample and total decay

C   the time taken for the radioactivity of a sample to decline by a factor of 2^x, where x is the number of half-lives having occurred

D   the time taken for half the atoms in a radioactive sample to decay

12   The diagram below has multiple structures labelled in the ear.

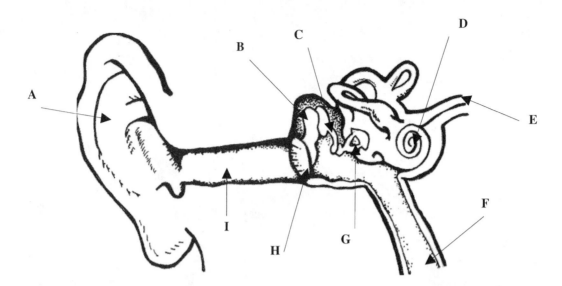

A sound wave arriving at the outer ear (structure **A**) becomes louder and higher pitched.

Which answer choice correctly describes the change in the displacement of the eardrum (structure **H**) when this occurs?

	Amplitude:	Frequency:	Direction:
A	increases	increases	longitudinal
B	decreases	increases	longitudinal
C	increases	increases	transverse
D	increases	decreases	transverse
E	decreases	decreases	longitudinal

13   In the figure below, two semicircles are inscribed in a square with sides of length x. If both semicircles have a diameter equal to the length of a side of the square, what is the area of the shaded region?

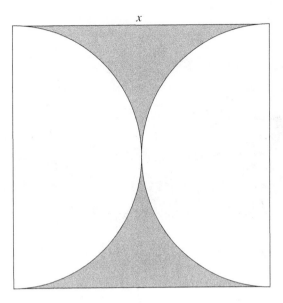

A $\dfrac{x^2(4-\pi)}{4}$

B $\dfrac{x^2}{\pi}$

C $\pi - \dfrac{x}{4}$

D πr^2

14 $2\,KI + Cl_2 \rightarrow 2\,KCl + I_2$

What is the best description of the above reaction?

A   Decomposition

B   Double Displacement Reaction

C   Single Displacement Reaction

D   Combustion

15   When a beam of white light enters a prism it is refracted and 'splits' into different colours bounded by two
      lines, a and b. The number of degrees of refraction is proportional to the wavelength of the light.

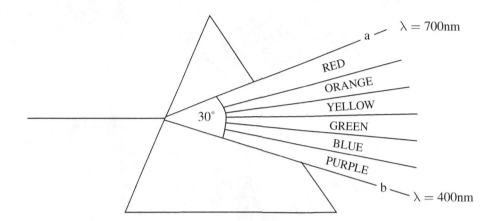

What is the frequency of the light that is refracted 10° below line a?

(All components of the electromagnetic spectrum travel at the speed of light, 3×108 m/s.)

A 5×10^5 Hz

B 5×10^{11} Hz

C 5×10^{14} Hz

D 6×10^{14} Hz

16   In some reptiles, reproduction is sexual, but the sex of the foetus is determined by the temperature of the
      environment at the time of fertilization.

      Which of the following features does this system definitely share with human sex selection?

      1   The sex cannot be predicted pre-fertilization.
      2   A 1:1 ratio of males to females is expected.
      3   Meiosis is required.

      A   1 only

      B   2 only

      C   3 only

      D   1 and 2

      E   1 and 3

      F   2 and 3

      G   1, 2 and 3

17   A cluster of 12,500 bacteria are exposed to an antibiotic at time 0 and just after 6 hours.

Bacteria that are not resistant have a 90% chance of immediate death, while 20% of the initial cluster of bacteria carry a gene which gives them complete resistance to the antibiotic.

The bacteria divide so that their numbers double in quantity every 6 hours.

What percentage of the bacteria are resistant to the antibiotic after 12 hours?

A   44%

B   47%

C   90%

D   96%

18   An exercise physiologist is performing an experiment to look at changes in breathing during exercise. He enlists a volunteer and has her pedal on an exercise bike while blowing into a tube. Her respiratory rate is measured with a strap on her chest, and all of the air that she breathes in and out is measured and plotted on the graph below, with positive values reflecting inhalation and negative values reflecting exhalation. As the woman begins pedalling from rest, what would you expect to happen to the data in the graph.

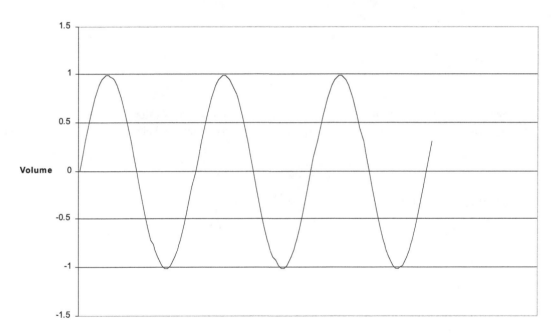

A   The frequency of the wave would decrease and the amplitude would decrease.

B   The frequency of the wave would decrease and the amplitude would increase.

C   The characteristics of the wave would not change.

D   The frequency of the wave would increase and the amplitude would decrease.

E   The frequency of the wave would increase and the amplitude would increase.

19 A compound in analysis is found to be composed of 40 % Carbon, 53.3 % Oxygen and 6.7 % Hydrogen by mass. Which of the following could be a chemical formula for this unknown compound?

A $C_2O_2H_8$

B $C_4O_2H_4$

C $C_4O_4H_4$

D $C_4O_4H_8$

20 If $a = \dfrac{b + x}{c + x}$ which of the following constant values for a, b and c will give the greatest value of x?

A $a = -2$ $b = -3$ $c = -6$

B $a = -10$ $b = -3$ $c = -3$

C $a = -4$ $b = -7$ $c = -2$

D $a = -2$ $b = -6$ $c = -3$

E $a = -4$ $b = -2$ $c = -7$

21 Approximately how long will it take a 3.00×10^6 kilowatt motor on an elevator to lift an elevator a distance of 40.0 m with three passengers if the combined mass of the passengers and elevator is 1.00 megagrams?

$g = 10$ m/s^2

A 0.00013 seconds

B 0.13 seconds

C 38 seconds

D 21 minutes and 40 seconds

22   Carbonic acid plays a critical buffering role in the blood.

$$CO_2 + H_2O \rightleftharpoons H_2CO_3 \rightleftharpoons H+ \ + HCO_{3-}$$

Which of the following will lower the pH from its normal value of 7.4?

    I   Breathing into a paper bag, thereby increasing the concentration of carbon dioxide in the blood.

    II   Adding another source of carbonate ions (HCO_{3-}) into the blood.

    III   Breathing pure oxygen.

A   I only

B   I and II

C   II and III

D   III only

E   I, II, and III

23   The molecular weight of chromium oxide is 152 g/mol. If approximately 32% of the mass of chromium oxide is provided by oxygen, what is the correct formula for chromium oxide? (Atomic weight of Cr = 52 and O = 16)

A Cr_3O_2

B Cr_2O_3

C CrO_2

D CrO_3

24   If the transformer below must supply 40 volts and 9 amps at the secondary coil, what must be provided to the primary coil?

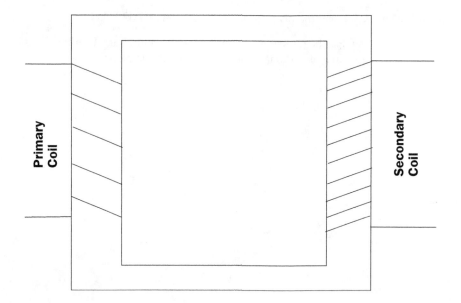

A   20 volts and 4.5 amps

B   20 volts and 18 amps

C   80 volts and 4.5 amps

D   80 volts and 18 amps

25   In the figure below, the length of segment PS is $2x + 12$, and the length of segment PQ is $6x - 10$. If R is the midpoint of segment QS, what is the length of segment PR?

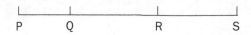

A $4x + 1$

B $2x + 22$

C $-2x + 22$

D $-2x + 11$

E $-4x + 22$

26   The beaker below contains a semi-permeable membrane separating two equal sized chambers, *A* and *B*. Each side has just been filled with a solution with a different concentration of solute X. Solute X cannot pass through the semi-permeable membrane, but water can. If the solution on side *A* initially contains a higher concentration of solute X then side *B*, how will the volumes change once equilibrium has been established?

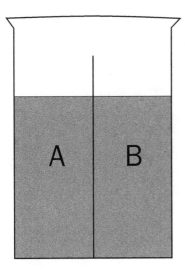

A   Volume *A* = Volume *B*

B   Volume *A* > Volume *B*

C   Volume *A* < Volume *B*

D   Cannot be determined

27   The following scheme represents a cycle of chemical reactions. J, L, M, Q and R represent individual chemical species.

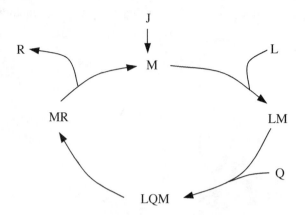

Which of the following best describes L, Q, M and LQM?

	L	Q	M	LQM
A	reagent	reagent	intermediate	product
B	reagent	catalyst	reagent	product
C	reagent	reagent	catalyst	intermediate
D	product	product	catalyst	reagent
E	intermediate	catalyst	reagent	intermediate

BMAT SECTION 3: WRITING TASK (30 MINUTES)

Section 3 contains a choice of three tasks. You have 30 minutes in which to answer **one**. You can take notes and make an outline in the space provided in the test booklet, but your answer must be written within the space provided on the answer sheet.

There is no correct answer to any of the questions posed. The writing task provides you with an opportunity to demonstrate your ability to:

- organise and develop your thoughts, and
- produce clear and concise written communication

Be sure to take time to organise your ideas and develop an outline. You may not use a dictionary but you may include a drawing or diagram.

Remember that you have only 30 minutes to select your task, organise your thoughts, and complete your essay.

USE THIS SPACE FOR NOTES

Answer <u>one</u> of the following questions.

1   **In an emergency, wherever it arises, you must offer assistance, taking account of your own safety, your competence, and the availability of other options for care.**

(UK General Medical Council, *Good Medical Practice 2009*)

Why must a doctor always offer assistance in an emergency? Under what circumstances is it acceptable for a doctor to limit that assistance? How can a doctor balance these concerns?

2   **It is irrational to regard the 'mind' as distinct from the body.**

What does the above statement mean? Provide examples of why it might be logical to distinguish the mind from the body and others that support the statement. Can you resolve the apparent contradiction?

3   **If the facts don't fit the theory, change the facts.**

(Albert Einstein)

Explain what you believe the author means by the above statement. How would you refute this statement? Do you believe that theories drive facts or that facts drive theories in contemporary scientific process?

BMAT TEST 1 – ANSWER KEY

SECTION 1	
Question	Answer
1	G
2	E
3	C
4	C
5	C
6	B
7	D
8	C
9	C
10	E
11	A
12	D
13	E
14	A
15	A
16	E
17	D
18	C
19	A
20	C
21	E
22	A
23	B
24	B
25	A
26	C
27	D
28	B
29	D
30	F
31	E
32	B
33	E
34	D
35	A

SECTION 2	
Question	Answer
1	A
2	D
3	A
4	A
5	A
6	C
7	B
8	A
9	B
10	D
11	B
12	A
13	A
14	C
15	C
16	C
17	D
18	E
19	D
20	E
21	A
22	A
23	B
24	B
25	A
26	B
27	C

BMAT TEST 1 – SCORING TABLES

1. Count up your number of correct answers in each section. Each question is worth one mark.

2. Write the total number of marks correct in each section on the lines below.

3. Find your approximate score for each section in the table below.

	NUMBER CORRECT	APPROXIMATE BMAT SCORE
Section 1	_____	_____
Section 2	_____	_____

SECTION 1		SECTION 2	
Number Correct	BMAT Score	Number Correct	BMAT Score
0	1.0	0	1.0
1	1.0	1	1.0
2	1.0	2	1.0
3	1.0	3	1.3
4	1.0	4	1.8
5	1.1	5	2.2
6	1.5	6	2.6
7	1.9	7	2.9
8	2.2	8	3.2
9	2.5	9	3.5
10	2.8	10	3.7
11	3.1	11	4.0
12	3.4	12	4.2
13	3.6	13	4.5
14	3.9	14	4.7
15	4.1	15	4.9
16	4.4	16	5.2
17	4.6	17	5.4
18	4.9	18	5.6
19	5.1	19	5.9
20	5.4	20	6.2
21	5.6	21	6.5
22	5.9	22	6.8
23	6.1	23	7.2
24	6.4	24	7.7
25	6.7	25	8.3
26	7.0	26	9.0
27	7.3	27	9.0
28	7.6		
29	8.0		
30	8.4		
31	8.9		
32	9.0		
33	9.0		
34	9.0		
35	9.0		

N.B. These scores are for approximation purposes only. The scoring tables used for the BMAT vary slightly year to year, depending on student performance and the norming of the questions in each version of the test paper. To err on the side of caution, these scoring tables are among the toughest ever used on the BMAT. In most cases, a similar performance on the BMAT would result in a slightly higher score.

Test 2

BMAT
Section 1

Test ID — Test 1 ○ Test 2 ● Test 3 ○

Last Name

First Name

Date

Completely fill in the space for your intended answer choice

A B C D E
○ ○ ● ○ ○

1 A B C D E
   ○ ○ ○ ○ ○

2 A B C D E F
   ○ ○ ○ ○ ○ ○

3 A B C D E
   ○ ○ ○ ○ ○

4 A B C D E
   ○ ○ ○ ○ ○

5 A B C D E
   ○ ○ ○ ○ ○

6 A B C D E
   ○ ○ ○ ○ ○

7 A B C D E
   ○ ○ ○ ○ ○

8 A B C D E F G H
   ○ ○ ○ ○ ○ ○ ○ ○

9 A B C D E
   ○ ○ ○ ○ ○

10 A B C D E
   ○ ○ ○ ○ ○

11 A B C D
   ○ ○ ○ ○

12 A B C D
   ○ ○ ○ ○

13 A B C D
   ○ ○ ○ ○

14 A B C D E F
   ○ ○ ○ ○ ○ ○

15 A B C D
   ○ ○ ○ ○

16 A B C D E
   ○ ○ ○ ○ ○

17 A B C D E
   ○ ○ ○ ○ ○

18 A B C D
   ○ ○ ○ ○

19 A B C D
   ○ ○ ○ ○

20 A B C D
   ○ ○ ○ ○

21 A B C D
   ○ ○ ○ ○

22 A B C D E
   ○ ○ ○ ○ ○

23 A B C D E
   ○ ○ ○ ○ ○

24 A B C D E
   ○ ○ ○ ○ ○

25 A B C D
   ○ ○ ○ ○

26 A B C D
   ○ ○ ○ ○

27 A B C D E
   ○ ○ ○ ○ ○

28 A B C D E F G H
   ○ ○ ○ ○ ○ ○ ○ ○

29 A B C D E
   ○ ○ ○ ○ ○

30 A B C D E
   ○ ○ ○ ○ ○

31 A B C D E
   ○ ○ ○ ○ ○

32 A B C D
   ○ ○ ○ ○

33 A B C D
   ○ ○ ○ ○

34 A B C D E F G H
   ○ ○ ○ ○ ○ ○ ○ ○

35 A B C D
   ○ ○ ○ ○

BMAT is a registered trademark of Cambridge Assessment, which neither sponsors nor endorses this product.

K   51

BMAT
Section 2

KAPLAN

TEST PREP

Test ID Test 1 ○ Test 2 ● Test 3 ○

Last Name
[ ]

First Name
[ ]

Date
[ ][ ] [ ][ ] [ ][ ][ ][ ]

Completely fill in the space for your intended answer choice

A B C D E
○ ○ ● ○ ○

1 A B C D
   ○ ○ ○ ○

2 A B C D
   ○ ○ ○ ○

3 A B C D
   ○ ○ ○ ○

4 A B C D
   ○ ○ ○ ○

5 A B C D
   ○ ○ ○ ○

6 A B C D E
   ○ ○ ○ ○ ○

7 A B C D
   ○ ○ ○ ○

8 A B C D
   ○ ○ ○ ○

9 A B C D
   ○ ○ ○ ○

10 A B C D
    ○ ○ ○ ○

11 A B C D
    ○ ○ ○ ○

12 A B C D E
    ○ ○ ○ ○ ○

13 A B C D
    ○ ○ ○ ○

14 A B C D E
    ○ ○ ○ ○ ○

15 A B C D E F
    ○ ○ ○ ○ ○ ○

16 A B C D
    ○ ○ ○ ○

17 A B C D
    ○ ○ ○ ○

18 A B C D E
    ○ ○ ○ ○ ○

19 A B C D E F
    ○ ○ ○ ○ ○ ○

20 A B C D
    ○ ○ ○ ○

21 A B C D E F G
    ○ ○ ○ ○ ○ ○ ○

22 A B C D E
    ○ ○ ○ ○ ○

23 A B C D E
    ○ ○ ○ ○ ○

24 A B C D
    ○ ○ ○ ○

25 A B C D E
    ○ ○ ○ ○ ○

26 A B C D E
    ○ ○ ○ ○ ○

27 A B C D E
    ○ ○ ○ ○ ○

K BMAT is a registered trademark of Cambridge Assessment, which neither sponsors nor endorses this product.

BMAT
Section 3

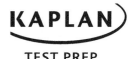

	Test 1	Test 2	Test 3	Test 4	Test 5	Test 6
Test ID	○	○	○	○	○	○

Last Name

First Name

Question answered

Your answer must be contained within this area.

BMAT is a registered trademark of Cambridge Assessment, which neither sponsors nor endorses this product.

K   53

BMAT SECTION 1: APTITUDE AND SKILLS (60 MINUTES)

You have 60 minutes to answer 35 questions. There are no penalties for incorrect answers, so you should attempt all questions.

Fill in your answers to each question on the answer sheet provided. Shade the circles corresponding to the answer choice(s) you have selected.

Avoid making stray marks on the paper. If you make a mistake, erase your answer completely and try again.

Calculators are **not** permitted.

1   Reducing class size in industrial countries has little effect, statistically speaking, on the education of the population. There are countries that have classes half the size, and their populations end up with more or less the same pass rates in examinations. Therefore arguments about class sizes in Britain's state education system are largely irrelevant to the education of the population.

Which one of the following is an underlying assumption of the above argument?

A   The cost of Britain's state education is disproportionate to its effectiveness.

B   Examination pass rates are a reliable measure of the education of the population.

C   Governments have a responsibility to organize efficient education services.

D   Advanced industrial countries have failed to improve the education of their inhabitants.

E   Reducing class size is the most effective of improving education.

2   Two cyclists are riding on a narrow cycle path through woodland. The total length of one circuit of the cycle path is 9 km. Shortly after starting the ride, the cyclist on the silver bike overtakes the cyclist on the yellow bike. The silver bike overtakes the yellow bike again later in the ride.

Both cyclists ride at a constant speed without stopping. The silver bike completes each circuit in 45 minutes and the yellow bike completes each circuit in 70 minutes.

How long after the first time does the silver bike overtake the yellow bike for the second time?

A   1 hour and 21 minutes

B   1 hour and 27 minutes

C   1 hour and 36 minutes

D   1 hour and 54 minutes

E   2 hours and 6 minutes

F   2 hours and 12 minutes

3   A school with students ages 6–16 years old has an enrolment of 700 students. 45% of the students are female, and 60% of the male students are under 10 years old. If 12 male students between the ages of 11–16 miss school one day, what percentage of male students between the ages of 11–16 are present that day? (to the nearest whole number)

    A   6%

    B   8%

    C   92%

    D   94%

    E   97%

4   Congestion on Italian roadways increased from 35% to 65% between 1982 and 1997. A typical solution to this problem has been to build more roadways, but studies have shown that building new roadways actually increases traffic by encouraging drivers to take longer trips and by making new destinations more available. Building new roadways also decreases the use of public transportation by promoting urban sprawl. Public funds should no longer be used for the construction of new roadways, but for the construction of better public transport systems.

    Which of the following are underlying assumptions of the above argument?

    1   Drivers are likely to be discouraged from taking long trips in the absence of new roadways.

    2   Most people prefer to drive than to take public transportation.

    3   Better public transportation is likely to alleviate some of the congestion on Italian roadways.

    A   1 only

    B   1 and 2 only

    C   3 only

    D   2 and 3 only

    E   1, 2, and 3

5 Five students are sitting in a row at the front of the classroom: Dylan, Katie, Sara, Colin and Fiona. Katie is sitting to the right of Colin, who is to the left of Sara. Fiona is to the left of Katie and to the right of Dylan.

Dylan must be left of:

A Katie and Fiona, but not necessarily Colin or Sara;

B Colin, but not necessarily Katie or Sara;

C Colin and Sara, but not necessarily Katie;

D Katie and Colin, but not necessarily Sara;

E Katie, Colin, and Sara.

6 Waleed painted a fresco using three 250 ml tubes of paint: one blue, one red and one yellow.

He mixed equal amounts of blue and red to make purple, equal amounts of yellow and red to make orange, equal amounts of blue and yellow to make green, and equal amounts of blue, red and yellow to make brown. Waleed mixes only the exact amounts of each colour required for the fresco.

The fresco consists of 25% yellow, 15% brown and 12% each of red, blue, purple, green and orange paint.

After mixing the paints and painting the fresco, Waleed has 40 ml of paint left in the yellow tube.

How much paint is left in the red tube?

A 90 ml

B 105 ml

C 120 ml

D 145 ml

E 160 ml

7   A group of physicists in the 1940s made three observations. First, life on Earth evolved very quickly. Second, there are about 100 billion stars in our galaxy. Third, an intelligent, exponentially reproducing extra-terrestrial species could easily colonise the galaxy in just a few million years. Putting these three facts together, they concluded that alien intelligence should by now be widespread. Enrico Fermi responded by asking: 'So, where is everybody?' In other words, if extra-terrestrial intelligence is common, isn't it unusual that we have never met a sentient species from another planet? The most plausible solution to this conundrum (known as Fermi's Paradox) is that highly evolved species self-destruct. If they are able to build a spaceship, they are also able to build weapons powerful enough to destroy all life on their planet, and sooner or later, unfortunately, such weapons always get used. Presumably the use of these weapons obliterates any trace of them or the species that created them, which is why the phenomenon cannot be observed.

Which one of the following is the best statement of the flaw in the above argument?

A   It asserts a theory that does not account for the wide range of evidence that disproves the theory.

B   It overlooks developments in astrophysics that have occurred since the 1940s.

C   It fails to specify what 'extra-terrestrial intelligence' entails.

D   It misinterprets the absence of evidence of a phenomenon as proof that alien species no longer exist.

E   It uses an example from science fiction to explain a real-life phenomenon that scientific experts have struggled to understand.

8   Speedy Cabs is a local minicab company with eight vehicles – four saloon cars and four estate cars, each a different colour. Each car is outfitted with a meter to record the total mileage travelled by the car since it was new.

The manager of the Speedy Cabs fleet records the mileage readings from the cars' meters at the end of the last day of every month. The table below indicates these readings for the first half of the year.

	January	February	March	April	May	June
White saloon	41 860	44 485	47 621	51 296	53 879	56 305
Silver saloon	56 191	59 348	61 214	65 981	69 305	72 023
Black saloon	79 783	82 061	84 154	86 247	91 793	94 528
Maroon saloon	68 332	70 906	73 398	77 461	81 317	85 462
Blue estate	49 106	52 941	55 047	58 289	62 893	64 038
Red estate	65 394	68 174	71 002	74 927	77 230	79 518
Grey estate	51 831	54 023	56 640	59 257	64 446	67 429
Green estate	60 458	63 019	67 835	70 043	72 981	74 507

Which car travelled the most miles during the three months from 1st March to 31st May?

A   White saloon   **E**   Blue estate

B   Silver saloon   **F**   Red estate

C   Black saloon   **G**   Grey estate

D   Maroon saloon   **H**   Green estate

Question 9 to 12 refer to the following information:

The chart below shows the number of visits per 1,000 men and 1,000 women in London to a major London Department Store. The chart shows the departments visited for men and women separately. The proportion of men and women in the population may be assumed to be the same.

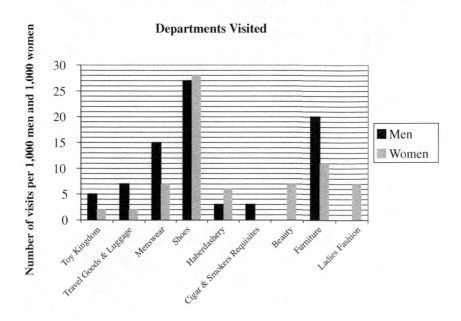

9   The percentage of men in London who visited the Travel Goods & Luggage Department was:

A   0.007%

B   0.07%

C   0.7%

D   7.0%

E   70.0%

10 Out of 10,000 people (men and women), how many visited the Shoe Department last week? (to the nearest whole number)

    A   55

    B   225

    C   275

    D   280

    E   550

11 If 1,200 men visited the store, how many shopped in the Menswear Department?

    A   150

    B   165

    C   180

    D   225

12 In which of the following pie charts is the proportion of departments visited by women correctly shown?

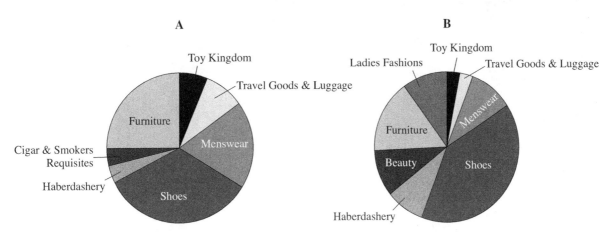

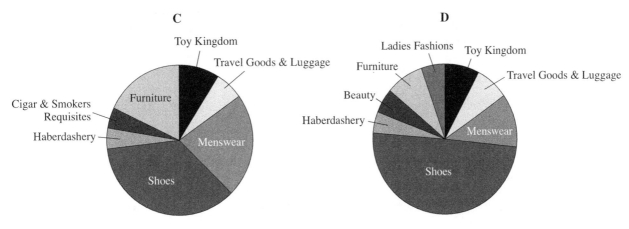

13   Each year, the number of accidents and injuries caused by speeding cars in the city centre rises. Thus the city council must impose a speed limit of 20 miles per hour on all roads in the city centre. Reducing the maximum speed of vehicles travelling through the city will surely lead to a reduction in accidents and injuries.

Which one of the following, if true, would most weaken the above argument?

A   The population of the city centre has decreased year-on-year for the last few years.

B   Most people who drive cars in the city centre do not live in the city.

C   A similar-sized city had more car accidents in the city centre after reducing the speed limit to 20 mph.

D   Most accidents and injuries in traffic collisions in the city centre are caused by trucks and lorries, not cars.

14   In the sport of Foeball, two types of goal can be scored: a deem, worth 8 points, and a wont, worth 3 points.

Last night, the Nobles played the Royals in Foeball. The Nobles won the match by 1 point.

    The Nobles scored one deem fewer than the Royals.

    The Royals scored exactly twice as many deems as wonts.

    The Nobles scored one more wont than deems.

How many wonts did the Nobles score in last night's match?

A   3

B   4

C   5

D   6

E   7

F   8

15   A recent study showed that women over 65 who took a class of antidepressants called SSRIs were at a 70% increased risk for a potentially disabling hip fracture than women who did not take antidepressants. The researchers have concluded that SSRIs lead to brittle bones.

Which one of the following is a reason why this conclusion might be unsafe?

A   The participants' hip fractures may have been caused by factors independent of the SSRIs.

B   Men over 70 do not experience as many hip fractures as women in the same age group.

C   Something in the medication other than the active SSRI ingredient may be responsible for the fractures.

D   If enough trials are carried out, some will show statistical significance purely by chance.

16   Students are devising ever-more ingenious ways to cheat in exams, thanks to modern technology. A common approach is to use a tiny earpiece along with a miniature wireless camera disguised as a button on the student's shirt. The student can then aim the camera at the test paper and wait for helpers outside the examination room to relay the answers via the earpiece. These cameras and earpieces can be difficult to detect unless you are trained to look for them. As with any approach to cheating, increased vigilance by teachers and invigilators is required. The best solution is to end the practice of having students take exams all in the same room. By separating students into individual rooms, they will not be able to copy each other's answers and they will never be sure if someone is watching at any particular moment.

Which of the following best expresses the flaw in the argument above?

A   It fails to consider the cost and staffing requirements of a new system of students taking exams in individual rooms.

B   It proposes a solution that does not address the problem of students cheating with the aid of new technologies.

C   It overlooks the reasons that students cheat in exams.

D   It assumes that teachers and invigilators will want to stop students from cheating in exams.

E   It asserts that technology can help students cheat in exams without providing evidence for this claim

17   The graph below shows the colour choices for new cars purchased last year.

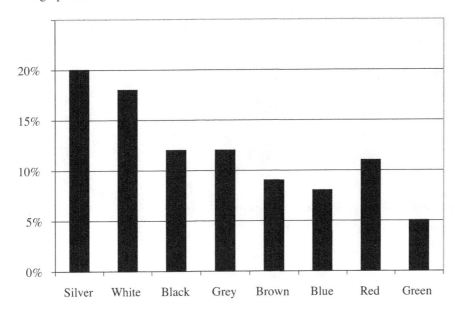

Which of the following statements can be deduced from the information provided?

1   A 30-year-old man was most likely to purchase a silver car.

2   A 23-year-old woman was most likely to purchase a car that was neither silver nor white.

3   A married couple shopping for a new car this year has a 50% chance of buying a car that is silver, white or black.

A   1 only   D   All

B   2 only   E   None

C   1 and 3 only

Questions 18 to 21 refer to the following information:

A video game contest is going on in two different rooms, the East Room and the West Room. Because of a malfunction, David is moved to the West Room to continue playing. The director notes that this will cause the average score to rise in the West Room whereas the average age there will decrease.

The contestants' scores and ages are shown in the table below in their positions before the move.

East Room				West Room			
Number	Name	Score	Age	Number	Name	Score	Age
1	George	150	10	7	Ahmed	150	14
2	David	250	6	8	Edward	160	12
3	Sara	270	12	9	Alistair	170	13
4	Louise	100	15	10	Caroline	210	14
5	Stephen	140	13	11	Meredith	260	15
6	Smeeta	200	14	12	Emma	220	10
	Total	1110			Total	1170	

18   What is the average age in the West Room after David's move?

A   11

B   12

C   13

D   14

19   By how much will the average score in the East Room change after David's move?

A   7

B   13

C   42

D   172

20   Which player is missing from this bar chart representing the scores of all the players?

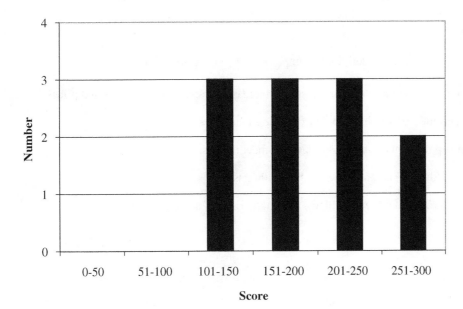

A   Louise

B   George

C   Meredith

D   Smeeta

21   A malfunction causes all players to get a 15% increase in their score. What is their total score?

A   2,447

B   2,456

C   2,622

D   2,736

22   The legalisation of marijuana has long been an issue. Those against legalisation argue that it will make marijuana more available and lead to an increase in marijuana consumption. Furthermore, marijuana is a "gateway drug" and increased marijuana consumption will lead to more dangerous and addictive drugs like cocaine and heroin.

Which one of the following is an underlying assumption of the above argument?

A   More children will use marijuana as a result of increased availability and decreased prices.

B   The law is currently preventing people from using marijuana.

C   The current supply of marijuana is sufficient to meet increased demand.

D   Marijuana is addictive and poses serious health threats.

E   Cocaine and heroin should remain illegal due to the risks of addiction and overdose.

23   A code breaker translates 'phe bult deng' into 'army moving west' and 'phe twalt fengu' into 'navy moving north.' Which of the following must be the word for army?

A   phe

B   bult

C   deng

D   phe or deng

E   bult or deng

24   For many years, topologists believed that snakes had no social life. Mother rattlesnakes, for instance, were thought to abandon their babies at birth. That evidence has been contradicted, however, by recent observations of rattlesnakes protecting their young from predators with as much ferocious commitment as any mammal parent. It would be going too far to conclude from this that snakes have the same bonding instincts as mammals, but we can say that they do have some kind of social life.

Which **one** of the following best summarises the main conclusion of the argument?

A   Old observations of rattlesnakes were not always accurate.

B   The social life of snakes is different from that of mammals.

C   Snakes bond with their young just like mammals do.

D   Recent evidence suggests that snakes have a social life.

E   Rattlesnakes love their young as much as mammals.

25   Brighton is 175 km from Oxford and 300 km from Cardiff. A train leaves from Cardiff traveling at 60 km/hr towards Brighton at the same time that a train leaves from Oxford traveling 75 km/hr. Assuming that the trains are traveling in a straight line, what is the time gap in minutes between the arrivals of the two trains?

    A   2 hours, 20 minutes

    B   2 hours, 40 minutes

    C   3 hours, 20 minutes

    D   5 hours

26   A bag contains 25 marbles: 12 blue, 6 black and 7 red. The first marble drawn out of the bag is red. What are the chances that the second marble drawn out of the bag will be red? (To the nearest percentage.)

    A   7%

    B   24%

    C   25%

    D   28%

27   Musical talent depends on aptitude – sensitivity to sounds and the proclivity to produce them – but ultimately, an individual's aptitude comes to nothing unless they have models to guide them in developing their talent into musical skills. This explains why all the great musicians were able to surpass their teachers, even when they had no family history of musical talent. Thus, if a student is to develop their talent for playing a musical instrument, they must listen to classical music, whether it's the radio, recordings or live orchestras.

Which one of the following best describes the flaw in the argument above?

    A   It fails to consider the role of parents and teachers in nurturing musical talent.

    B   It assumes that anyone who listens to classical music will develop into a classical musician without providing evidence for this claim.

    C   It ignores the possibility that classical music may not model the skills required for other types of music, such as rock or jazz.

    D   It assumes that musical success depends on having parents or teachers who can guide you in the early stages of a musical career.

    E   It ignores the views of classical musicians who achieved success despite not being able to attend a live orchestra in their formative years.

28   A game called Quintris is played with a series of different pieces each consisting of 5 squares. There are only certain pieces available in Quintris, though each piece can be rotated clockwise any number of times.

The goal of Quintris is to rotate each new piece so it slots into any gaps in the playing field. Each new piece appears at the top of the playing field; you must rotate it and shift it into position before it falls to the bottom. The playing field is indicated by the thick lines in the diagram below.

Once all the squares in a row are filled, the row will disappear from the playing field, which causes all the blocks in incomplete rows above to shift down the playing field.

A partially completed game of Quintris is shown in the diagram. A Quintris player would like to fill the gap and remove the bottom four rows of the diagram with her next two Quintris pieces.

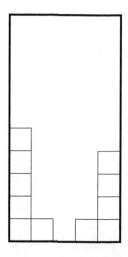

Which one of the following pairs could be the missing pieces that would complete the bottom four rows?

A

B

C

D

E

F

G

H

29   I have two different bankcards, each with a unique four-digit PIN. All but one of the digits from 1 to 9 appears in one of my PINs. The four digits in each PIN add up to 21.

Which non-zero digit appears in neither of the two PINs?

A   1

B   3

C   5

D   7

E   9

30   Last year's fundraising luncheon raised just over £20 000, and the budget committee should assume that we will raise at least that much at this year's event. We have already matched last year's level of corporate sponsorship, with 70% of the companies from last year pledging donations again this year. Even more exciting, more than 45% of the individuals to whom invitations were sent have purchased tickets, whereas last year, only 20% of those invited bought tickets. The ticket price is exactly same as last year.

The argument above is questionable because it takes for granted which one of the following?

A   The budget committee has not already concluded that the luncheon will raise more than £20 000.

B   Individual donations (through the purchase of tickets) will rise more this year than corporate sponsorship.

C   70% of last year's corporate sponsors will collectively donate as much this year as 100% did last year.

D   There will be exactly 25% more invited individuals in attendance this year than there were last year.

E   An increase in the percentage of ticket purchasers rules out the possibility of a decrease in the number of ticket purchasers.

31   The Belleville Hotel charges for bed and breakfast based on the length of your stay at the hotel.

first three nights   -   €90 per night

fourth and subsequent nights   -   €80 per night

If a guest stays for eight or more consecutive nights, they pay €80 per night for the entire stay at the hotel.

The hotel bill will also include the charges for using the hotel car park. The hotel car park costs €8 per night or €20 for a three-night parking pass. Louise will always pay for the parking pass if it works out to be cheaper than paying per night for the car park.

Louise stayed at the hotel last month for six consecutive nights, keeping her car in the hotel car park. She has booked ten consecutive nights at the hotel next month, and she will keep her car in the hotel car park once again. Louise never has any other charges added to her hotel bill.

How much more than last month will Louise's bill for next month's stay at the Belleville Hotel be?

A   €268

B   €298

C   €318

D   €348

E   €378

Questions 32 to 35 refer to the following information:

In 2017, debit card payments overtook cash as the most common type of transaction in the UK. UK customers used debit cards 13.2 billion times in 2017, a rise of 14% from the previous year, whilst cash was used in 13.1 billion transactions in 2017, down 15% from the previous year. Despite the decline in cash purchases, cash accounted for 34% of all transactions in the UK in 2017, and 2.2 million customers use cash for all their day-to-day purchases. At the same time, 63% of people in the UK had at least one contactless card, and 3.4 million people in the UK never use cash, always relying on cards.

As more people rely on debit cards and contactless payments, it is projected that cash will only make up 6.5 billion transactions, or 16% of the total for the UK, by 2027, falling below 10% by the mid-2030s. There is a real risk that a significant number of people in the UK who continue to rely on cash by then will find it difficult to cope, as many retailers may stop taking cash payments. A recent study found that as many as 17% of adults would struggle to get by in a cashless society.

The greatest risk to those adults depending on cash transactions is the number of ATMs in the UK, which is dropping at a worrying rate. Currently ATMs are being shut down at a rate of 300 a month. As a result, people in smaller towns and rural areas may have to travel some distance to find an ATM, adding to the cost and difficulty of using cash.

The value of banknotes issued by the Bank of England in circulation has risen by 22.5% from 2014 to 2018, suggesting that our reliance on cash has not abated with the increased use of debit cards. However, the year-on-year increase was relatively low from 2017 to 2018, suggesting a slowing trend as cash starts to fall out of favour.

Value of banknotes issued by the Bank of England in circulation (in millions of pounds)

	£5	£10	£20	£50	Total
2014	1,540	7,182	36,483	11,025	56,230
2015	1,601	7,371	38,912	11,788	59,671
2016	1,645	7,767	41,037	13,157	63,606
2017	1,912	8,006	43,357	15,601	68,876
2018	1,910	7,789	42,692	16,508	68,899

Value of new banknotes issued by the Bank of England (in millions of pounds)

	£5	£10	£20	£50	Total
2013	793	2,141	5,281	2,260	10,474
2014	869	2,433	6,202	2,165	11,668
2015	977	5,683	5,056	1,831	13,547
2016	1,643	4,008	6,382	3,188	15,220
2017	386	8,192	3,291	2,169	14,039

Value of banknotes destroyed by the Bank of England (in millions of pounds)

	£5	£10	£20	£50	Total
2013	927	2,811	3,821	1,874	9,432
2014	1,001	2,351	3,848	1,739	8,939
2015	893	5,250	3,547	481	10,172
2016	1,509	4,058	3,371	484	9,422
2017	1,192	7,785	3,474	506	12,956

32 How many more £20 notes than £50 notes were in circulation in 2018?

A 1,804,440,000

B 1,855,830,000

C 2,568,700,000

D 2,618,400,000

33 What greater value of new £5 notes were put into circulation in 2016 as compared to 2015?

A 64.3%

B 65.4%

C 66.7%

D 68.2%

34 Which of the following statements can be concluded from the information in the tables and the text?

1 The Bank of England destroyed 27% fewer £50 notes in 2017 as compared to 5 years earlier.

2 Cash transactions in the UK are projected to decline by more than 50% over ten years.

3 Most new banknotes issued by the Bank of England in 2017 were £10 notes.

A 1 only

B 2 only

C 3 only

D 1 and 2 only

E 1 and 3 only

F 2 and 3 only

G 1, 2 and 3

H none of them

35 What proportional value of banknotes destroyed in 2017 were £10 notes?

A £1.75 of every £3

B £3 of every £5

C £1.25 of every £2

D £2.75 of every £4

BMAT SECTION 2: SCIENTIFIC KNOWLEDGE AND APPLICATIONS (30 MINUTES)

You have 30 minutes to answer 27 questions. There are no penalties for incorrect answers, so you should attempt all questions.

Fill in your answers to each question on the answer sheet provided. Shade the circles corresponding to the answer choice(s) you have selected.

Avoid making stray marks on the paper. If you make a mistake, erase your answer completely and try again.

Calculators are **not** permitted.

1   Which part of a nerve cell releases neurotransmitter?

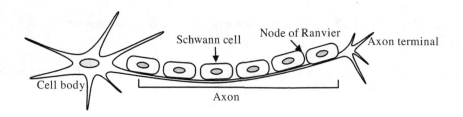

A   Cell body

B   Axon

C   Axon terminal

D   Node of Ranvier

2   Which of the following circuits has the greatest total equivalent resistance?

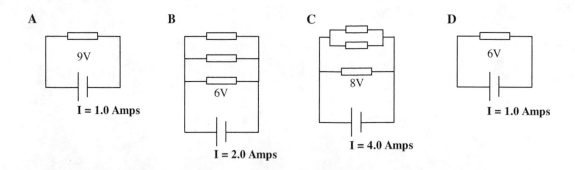

3   Which row of the table does NOT give an appropriate tool for making a diagnosis of the condition given?

	Condition	Equipment
A	myocardial infarction (heart attack)	ECG
B	asthma	Peak Expiratory Flow meter
C	bacterial infection	white blood cell level
D	Type 2 diabetes	blood insulin level

4   The element $^{244}_{94}$Pu undergoes a series of radioactive decays and achieves a stable structure with an electron number of 92.

Which of the following decay chains could have occurred?

A   a series of 2 alpha decays with gamma release

B   a series of 1 alpha decay and 2 beta decays

C   a series of 2 beta decays with gamma release

D   a series of 2 alpha decays followed by 2 beta decays

5   For the quadratic equation $x^2 - 3x - 18 = 0$, which of the following statements is true?

A   The product of the roots is positive, and the sum of the roots is 3.

B   The product of the roots is negative, and the sum of the roots is 3.

C   The product of the roots is 0, and the sum of the roots is –6.

D   The product of the roots is negative, and the sum of the roots is –3.

6   Two elements from the same group of the periodic table have the electron configurations detailed below:

(i)   2, 7
(ii)   2, 8, 7

Which of the following statements is true about these elements? Select all that apply.

1   Element (ii) forms a 1^- ion more readily than element (i).

2   Element (ii) will displace ions of element (i) from aqueous solution.

3   These elements readily undergo reduction.

4   Element (ii) is a poisonous green gas at room temperature and pressure.

5   Element (i) has a lower melting point than element (ii).

A   1, 2 and 4

B   1, 3 and 4

C   2, 3 and 4

D   2, 4 and 5

E   3, 4 and 5

7   What is the area of the unshaded region?

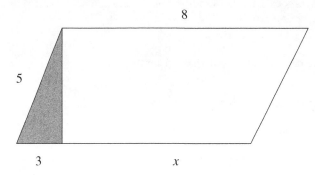

    A   22

    B   26

    C   32

    D   36

8   165 grams of $Pb(NO_3)_2$ (lead nitrate) is mixed with 152 grams of $FeSO_4$ (iron sulfate). How much $PbSO_4$ (lead sulfate) is produced in grams? The atomic weights are as follows: Pb, 207 g; N, 14 g; O, 16 g; Fe, 56 g; S, 32 g.

    A   151.5 g

    B   165.5 g

    C   303 g

    D   330 g

9   As part of an emissions test, a car is placed on a 'car treadmill' travelling at a constant speed of x m/s. The driver of the car is instructed to brake at a certain time.

The graph shows the velocity of the car with time. The time at which the driver is instructed to brake is shown with an arrow.

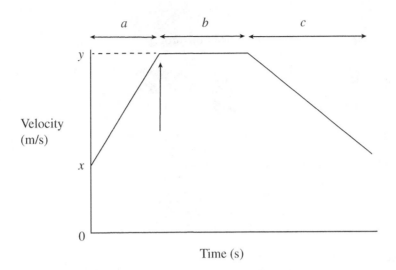

Which of the following is an expression for the *stopping distance* of the car in metres?

A $by + \dfrac{1}{2}c(x + y)$

B $by + \dfrac{1}{2}(x + y)(a + c)$

C $\dfrac{1}{2}(2b + c)(y - x)$

D $bc(x + y)$

10   The following statements are about stem cells.

1   Human embryonic stem cells have 23 pairs of chromosomes.

2   A stem cell from adult bone marrow could become a heart tissue cell.

3   An embryonic stem cell could become a heart tissue cell.

Which of the statements are correct?

A   1 and 2

B   1 and 3

C   2 and 3

D   1, 2 and 3

11 Hydrogen gas is reacted with iodine gas to form hydrogen iodide in an enclosed container.

$$H_2 (g) + I_2 (g) \rightleftharpoons 2HI (g)$$

The forward reaction is exothermic.

Which of the following would increase the yield of hydrogen iodide?

A   reducing the temperature of the system

B   increasing the volume of the container

C   increasing the pressure in the container

D   the addition of a catalyst

12 The reactions

(i) $(CH_3)_2C{=}O \rightarrow (CH_3)_2CHOH$
(ii) $2NO_3^- + 10e^- + 12 H^+ \rightarrow N_2 + 6H_2O$
(iii) $CO_2 + water + light\ energy \rightarrow C_6H_{12}O_6 + oxygen$

are all examples of:

A   organic synthesis

B   reduction

C   oxidation

D   displacement

E   photosynthesis

13   Submarines use sonar (sound waves) as a way of measuring distance or depth. In order to measure the distance from an enemy submarine, the sub sends out a sound wave (a 'ping') and 'hears' an echo 3 sec later. Approximately how far is the enemy sub if the speed of sound in water is 1320 m/sec?

A   0.5 km

B   1.3 km

C   2.0 km

D   4.0 km

14   A student is investigating the amount of force (F) used to jump into the air. She considers the maximum height of her jump and formulates the equation

$$0 = \frac{2(F-W)c}{\frac{W}{g}} - 2gH$$

Which of the following is a correct expression of F ?

A $W\left(1+\dfrac{H}{2c}\right)$

B $\dfrac{gH}{c} - W$

C $W\left(1+\dfrac{H}{c}\right)$

D $\dfrac{g\left(\dfrac{1}{W}+H\right)}{c}$

E $\dfrac{gH}{c} + W$

15   The chart below demonstrates a wave with a wavelength of 2 m. Each tick mark on the *x*-axis represents 1 sec; the *y*-axis is in metres.

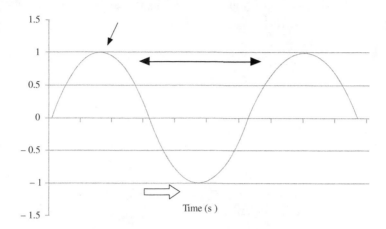

What is the speed of the wave?

A $\frac{1}{2}$ m/sec

B $\frac{1}{3}$ m/sec

C $\frac{2}{3}$ m/sec

D   2 m/sec

E   6 m/sec

F   Can not be determined uniquely from the information given

16 The following graph shows the gravitational potential energy gained with height lifted by a cube of surface area 13.5 m².

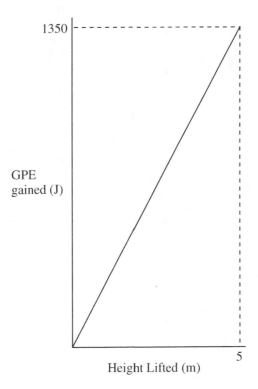

What is the density of the cube?

(Assume $g = 10$ m/s²)

A   0.12 kg/m³

B   2 kg/m³

C   5 kg/m³

D   8 kg/m³

17 The human immunodeficiency virus (HIV) infects immune system cells known as CD4⁺ T cells. These cells are responsible for initiating the immune response when the body is attacked by foreign invaders. Without these cells the host becomes susceptible to many types of infection. Which of the following is likely to be the least useful indicator of HIV infection progression?

A   HIV viral load

B   CD4⁺ cell count

C   presence of opportunistic infections

D   blood pressure

18   The graph shows the rate at which water is flowing in and out of a circular cylinder. Initially, the canister is empty.

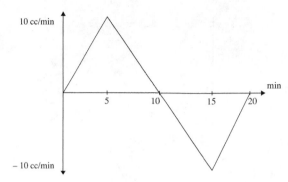

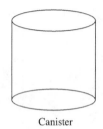

Canister

Which **one** of the following is true?

A   The canister is empty after 10 minutes.

B   The maximum volume of water in the canister is 10 cc.

C   At the 5-minute mark, the volume of water in the canister is 50 cc.

D   At the 5-minute mark, the volume of water in the canister is 25 cc.

E   Between the 5- and 10-minute mark, water is leaving the canister at a rate of 2 cc/min.

19 When isopropyl alcohol is burned in the presence of oxygen, it produces carbon dioxide and water.

The equation for this reaction is:

m C_3H_7OH + **n** O_2 → **p** CO_2 + **q** H_2O

What is the value of **q**?

A   4

B   6

C   8

D   9

E   12

F   15

20 A baseball with mass 200 g is traveling at 10 m/sec. It collides (an elastic collision) with cricket ball initially at rest, that then moves with a velocity of 5 m/sec. If the baseball has a velocity after the collision of 2 m/sec, what is the mass of the cricket ball?

A   240 g

B   267 g

C   320 g

D   400 g

21 Which of the following are major sources of background radiation?

1   Food and drink

2   Krypton gas

3   Cosmic rays

A   1 only

B   2 only

C   3 only

D   1 and 2

E   1 and 3

F   2 and 3

G   All

22   The structure of a short section of polymer is shown below:

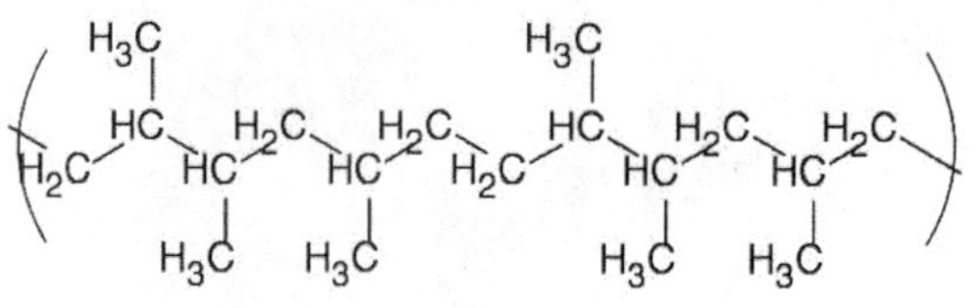

Which of the following could be the formula of its monomer?

A

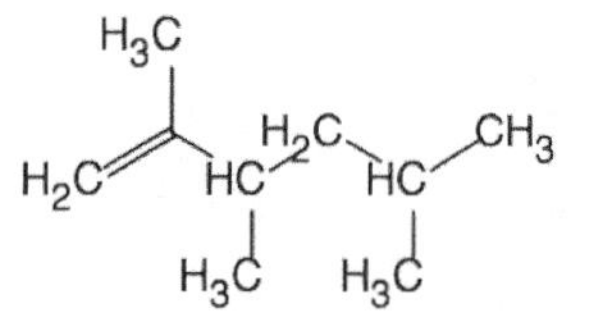

B

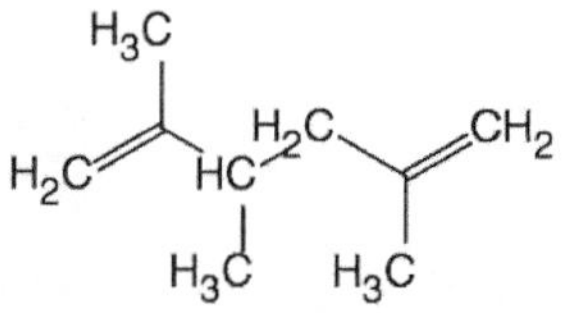

C

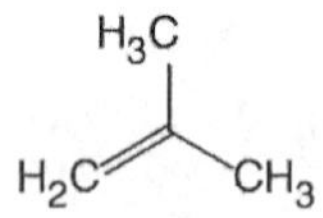

D

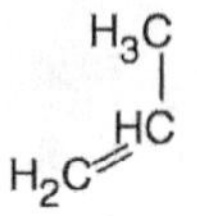

E

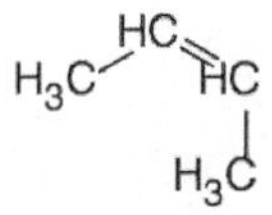

23   An accessory digestive organ is an organ that helps with digestion that is not a part of the digestive tract itself.

Which of the following are all accessory digestive organs?

A	salivary glands	oesophagus	gallbladder
B	vermiform appendix	teeth	anus
C	liver	pancreas	gallbladder
D	teeth	tongue	spleen
E	liver	gallbladder	small intestine

24   A new surgical technique is developed that has a failure rate of 0.5%. If the previously used technique had a failure rate of 1.5%, how many fewer surgical failures would there be in 10,000 patients who undergo the new procedure?

       A   75

       B   100

       C   125

       D   150

25   C is the center of the circle. ∠ABC is 70°. The radius of the circle is 18. What is the length of arc AB?

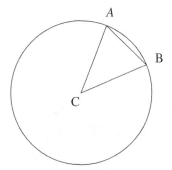

       A $\dfrac{\pi}{9}$

       B $\dfrac{2\pi}{9}$

       C 2π

       D 4π

       E 36π

26   A student is using a volumetric pipette to titrate a solution of H_2SO_4. The pipette volume is reported as 1.00 mL, and the titration requires 12 pipette volumes of KOH solution to neutralise 1 pipette volume of H_2SO_4 solution.

If the KOH solution concentration is reported as 0.100 moldm^{-3}, which of the following is an expression for is the maximum possible concentration (in moldm^{-3}) of the solution of H_2SO_4 that can be calculated from this data?

A $\dfrac{6 \times 1.005 \times 0.1000}{0.995}$

B $\dfrac{12 \times 0.995 \times 0.0995}{1.005}$

C $\dfrac{6 \times 0.995 \times 0.0995}{1.005}$

D $\dfrac{12 \times 1.005 \times 0.1005}{0.995}$

E $\dfrac{6 \times 1.005 \times 0.1005}{0.995}$

27   For the equation $y + 3 = (x - 4)^{\frac{2}{3}}$, what is the value of y if $x = 31$?

A   3

B   4

C   6

D   9

E   27

BMAT SECTION 3: WRITING TASK (30 MINUTES)

Section 3 contains a choice of three tasks. You have 30 minutes in which to answer **one**. You can take notes and make an outline in the space provided in the test booklet, but your answer must be written within the space provided on the answer sheet.

There is no correct answer to any of the questions posed. The writing task provides you with an opportunity to demonstrate your ability to:

- organise and develop your thoughts
- produce clear and concise written communication

Be sure to take time to organise your ideas and develop an outline. You may not use a dictionary but you may include a drawing or diagram.

Remember that you have only 30 minutes to select your task, organise your thoughts, and complete your essay.

Answer <u>one</u> of the following questions:

1   **Physicians make the worst patients.**

       What do you understand the above statement to mean? Provide examples of why physicians might sometimes make bad patients and other times make good patients. What does this analysis suggest about physicians' compassion toward their patients?

2   **No science is immune to the infection of politics and the corruption of power.**

       (Jacob Bronowski)

       What does the author mean by this statement? Develop an argument for an opposite position. How can you reconcile the two positions?

3   **The knowledge of the world is only to be acquired in the world, and not in a closet.**

       (Lord Chesterfield)

       Explain what the author means by the above statement. Can you suggest examples of ways in which education benefits from being sheltered from the world? What should be the balance between university training and practical experience in preparing for professional life?

BMAT TEST 2 – ANSWER KEY

SECTION 1	
Question	Answer
1	B
2	E
3	C
4	C
5	A
6	B
7	D
8	G
9	C
10	C
11	D
12	B
13	C
14	D
15	A
16	B
17	B
18	B
19	B
20	A
21	C
22	B
23	E
24	D
25	B
26	C
27	C
28	F
29	B
30	E
31	C
32	A
33	D
34	F
35	B

SECTION 2	
Question	Answer
1	C
2	C
3	D
4	D
5	B
6	E
7	B
8	A
9	A
10	B
11	A
12	B
13	C
14	C
15	B
16	D
17	D
18	D
19	C
20	C
21	E
22	D
23	C
24	B
25	D
26	E
27	C

K

BMAT TEST 2 – SCORING TABLES

1. Count up your number of correct answers in each section. Each question is worth one mark.

2. Write the total number of marks correct in each section on the lines below.

3. Find your approximate score for each section in the table below.

	NUMBER CORRECT	APPROXIMATE BMAT SCORE
Section 1	_____	_____
Section 2	_____	_____

SECTION 1		SECTION 2	
Number Correct	BMAT Score	Number Correct	BMAT Score
0	1.0	0	1.0
1	1.0	1	1.0
2	1.0	2	1.0
3	1.0	3	1.3
4	1.0	4	1.8
5	1.1	5	2.2
6	1.5	6	2.6
7	1.9	7	2.9
8	2.2	8	3.2
9	2.5	9	3.5
10	2.8	10	3.7
11	3.1	11	4.0
12	3.4	12	4.2
13	3.6	13	4.5
14	3.9	14	4.7
15	4.1	15	4.9
16	4.4	16	5.2
17	4.6	17	5.4
18	4.9	18	5.6
19	5.1	19	5.9
20	5.4	20	6.2
21	5.6	21	6.5
22	5.9	22	6.8
23	6.1	23	7.2
24	6.4	24	7.7
25	6.7	25	8.3
26	7.0	26	9.0
27	7.3	27	9.0
28	7.6		
29	8.0		
30	8.4		
31	8.9		
32	9.0		
33	9.0		
34	9.0		
35	9.0		

N.B. These scores are for approximation purposes only. The scoring tables used for the BMAT vary slightly year to year, depending on student performance and the norming of the questions in each version of the test paper. To err on the side of caution, these scoring tables are among the toughest ever used on the BMAT. In most cases, a similar performance on the BMAT would result in a slightly higher score.

Test 3

BMAT
Section 1

KAPLAN
TEST PREP

Test ID Test 1 ○ Test 2 ○ Test 3 ●

Last Name

First Name

Date

Completely fill in the space for your intended answer choice

A B C D E
○ ○ ● ○ ○

1 A B C D E
   ○ ○ ○ ○ ○

2 A B C D E F
   ○ ○ ○ ○ ○ ○

3 A B C D E F G H
   ○ ○ ○ ○ ○ ○ ○ ○

4 A B C D
   ○ ○ ○ ○

5 A B C D E
   ○ ○ ○ ○ ○

6 A B C D E
   ○ ○ ○ ○ ○

7 A B C D E F G
   ○ ○ ○ ○ ○ ○ ○

8 A B C D E
   ○ ○ ○ ○ ○

9 A B C D E F G H
   ○ ○ ○ ○ ○ ○ ○ ○

10 A B C D
   ○ ○ ○ ○

11 A B C D
   ○ ○ ○ ○

12 A B C D
   ○ ○ ○ ○

13 A B C D E
   ○ ○ ○ ○ ○

14 A B C D E F
   ○ ○ ○ ○ ○ ○

15 A B C D E
   ○ ○ ○ ○ ○

16 A B C D E
   ○ ○ ○ ○ ○

17 A B C D E
   ○ ○ ○ ○ ○

18 A B C D E F
   ○ ○ ○ ○ ○ ○

19 A B C D E
   ○ ○ ○ ○ ○

20 A B C D E F G H
   ○ ○ ○ ○ ○ ○ ○ ○

21 A B C D E
   ○ ○ ○ ○ ○

22 A B C D
   ○ ○ ○ ○

23 A B C D
   ○ ○ ○ ○

24 A B C D E F G H
   ○ ○ ○ ○ ○ ○ ○ ○

25 A B C D E
   ○ ○ ○ ○ ○

26 A B C D
   ○ ○ ○ ○

27 A B C D E
   ○ ○ ○ ○ ○

28 A B C D E F
   ○ ○ ○ ○ ○ ○

29 A B C D E
   ○ ○ ○ ○ ○

30 A B C D E
   ○ ○ ○ ○ ○

31 A B C D E
   ○ ○ ○ ○ ○

32 A B C D
   ○ ○ ○ ○

33 A B C D
   ○ ○ ○ ○

34 A B C D
   ○ ○ ○ ○

35 A B C D
   ○ ○ ○ ○

BMAT is a registered trademark of Cambridge Assessment, which neither sponsors nor endorses this product.

97

BMAT
Section 2

KAPLAN
TEST PREP

Test ID

Test 1	Test 2	Test 3
○	○	●

Last Name

First Name

Date

Completely fill in the space for your intended answer choice

A B C D E
○ ○ ● ○ ○

1 A B C D
   ○ ○ ○ ○

2 A B C D E
   ○ ○ ○ ○ ○

3 A B C D
   ○ ○ ○ ○

4 A B C D E F G
   ○ ○ ○ ○ ○ ○ ○

5 A B C D E
   ○ ○ ○ ○ ○

6 A B C D
   ○ ○ ○ ○

7 A B C D E
   ○ ○ ○ ○ ○

8 A B C D
   ○ ○ ○ ○

9 A B C D
   ○ ○ ○ ○

10 A B C D
    ○ ○ ○ ○

11 A B C D
    ○ ○ ○ ○

12 A B C D E
    ○ ○ ○ ○ ○

13 A B C D
    ○ ○ ○ ○

14 A B C D E
    ○ ○ ○ ○ ○

15 A B C D
    ○ ○ ○ ○

16 A B C D
    ○ ○ ○ ○

17 A B C D E
    ○ ○ ○ ○ ○

18 A B C D
    ○ ○ ○ ○

19 A B C D
    ○ ○ ○ ○

20 A B C D E
    ○ ○ ○ ○ ○

21 A B C D
    ○ ○ ○ ○

22 A B C D E F
    ○ ○ ○ ○ ○ ○

23 A B C D
    ○ ○ ○ ○

24 A B C D
    ○ ○ ○ ○

25 A B C D
    ○ ○ ○ ○

26 A B C D
    ○ ○ ○ ○

27 A B C D E
    ○ ○ ○ ○ ○

BMAT
Section 3

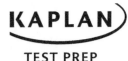

Test ID

	Test 1 ○	Test 2 ○	Test 3 ○	Test 4 ○	Test 5 ○	Test 6 ○

Last Name

First Name

Question answered

Your answer must be contained within this area.

BMAT is a registered trademark of Cambridge Assessment, which neither sponsors nor endorses this product.

99

BMAT SECTION 1: APTITUDE AND SKILLS (60 MINUTES)

You have 60 minutes to answer 35 questions. There are no penalties for incorrect answers, so you should attempt all questions.

Fill in your answers to each question on the answer sheet provided. Shade the circles corresponding to the answer choice(s) you have selected.

Avoid making stray marks on the paper. If you make a mistake, erase your answer completely and try again.

Calculators are **not** permitted.

1   The pie chart below represents the population of people suffering from heart disease.

Heart Disease Sufferers

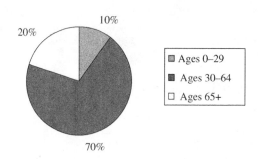

Which of the following conclusions can be logically drawn from the information in the chart above?

1   The risk of heart disease drops after the age of 65.

2   Heart disease is generally most severe in middle age.

3   Most people suffering from heart disease are neither very old nor very young.

A   1 and 3 only

B   2 and 3 only

C   3 only

D   All

E   None

2   A teacher is booking hotel rooms for a class trip. The group requires rooms for 18 students – with equal numbers of boys and girls – and four teachers. The prices per room are as follows:

Single: £55   Double: £80   Suite: £140 (up to 4 people per suite)

Special offers:
- £15 off each double room (if three or more double rooms are booked)
- £10 off each single room (if four or more single rooms are booked)

Boys must only share rooms with boys and girls must only share rooms with girls. The teachers may share rooms with each other but not with students, and all the teachers may not be booked into the same room.

What is the total cost of the rooms, applying any special offers, if they book the cheapest option?

A   £690

B   £735

C   £760

D   £795

E   £830

F   £875

3 I take a long piece of string and stretch it out into a straight line at full length. Then I make a small mark in the exact middle of the string with a thin purple felt-tip pen.

Next, I fold the string in half, holding onto both new ends and stretching it tight. This time, I use a thin black pen to make a small mark in the middle of each strand of the folded string.

After that, I fold it in half once again, this time using a thin red pen to make a mark in the middle of each strand of the folded string.

Then I fold it in half one final time and make a small green mark in the middle of each strand of the folded string.

Finally, I unfold the string and stretch it out to its original full length.

How many marks are there on the string between the red marks that are nearest to the ends of the string?

A   6

B   7

C   8

D   9

E   10

F   11

G   12

H   13

4 Guidelines for nutrition should reduce the suggested amount of carbohydrates in the average person's diet. A study has shown that when an obese person decreases carbohydrate consumption by twenty percent, the long-term result is a lower body fat ratio. Therefore, guidelines for carbohydrate consumption should be decreased by twenty percent.

Which **one** of the following, if true, would most **weaken** the argument above?

A   Many healthy athletes already consume twenty to thirty percent fewer carbohydrates than suggested by the guidelines.

B   Most of the study participants were consuming twice as many carbohydrates as recommended by the current guidelines prior to the study.

C   The study did not distinguish between the types of carbohydrates consumed.

D   A high protein diet has been found to be the quickest way to lose fat.

5   A political candidate has publicly claimed on several occasions that legislation protecting air quality is a laudable goal. She has also said that air quality in her district is an increasingly important public health issue. In a recent interview, however, the candidate said that, if elected, she would not support such legislation. We can not put our trust in someone who contradicts herself so blatantly.

Which one of the following is taken for granted in the argument above?

A   The candidate will not support the legislation.

B   The candidate is not otherwise trustworthy.

C   The candidate did not change her mind after giving the interview.

D   If something is a laudable goal, it is an important health issue.

E   If something is a laudable goal, it should be supported.

6   One of the games at the school fete was 'Guess How Many Sweets are in the Jar.' Prizes were given based on how close each person guessed to the exact number. The top five prizes are shown in the table.

Prize	Guess	Winner
1st	352	Laura
2nd	391	Amir
3rd	395	Michelle
4th	346	Evan
5th	343	Sophie

How many sweets were in the jar?

A   368

B   369

C   370

D   371

E   372

7   A school has 300 students, in five year groups. The table below provides some information about the numbers of girls and boys in each year group.

Year	Girls	Boys	Total
7	26		62
8		17	59
9			
10			59
11		12	56
Total		120	300

There is a probability of 1 in 5 that a girl selected at random is in Year 9.

What is the probability that a Year 9 student selected at random is a girl?

A   3 in 8

B   2 in 5

C   7 in 16

D   1 in 2

E   9 in 16

F   3 in 5

G   11 in 16

8   It was Charles Darwin who first divided taxonomists into 'lumpers' and 'splitters.' The first group tends to see similarities, fitting lots of animals together into broad categories. The second group is more likely to particularise, dividing things up based on minor variations. The botanist who created A. *Bulbophyllum* (the largest orchid genus) was clearly a lumper. He put over 1,500 species into this single genus. It now has over 1,800 accepted species.

What is the conclusion of the argument above?

A   The scientist who created A. *Bulbophyllum* was a lumper.

B   Charles Darwin divided taxonomists into two broad categories.

C   It is suspicious that the genus A. *Bulbophyllum* has 1,500 species in it.

D   Lumpers tend to be more optimistic than splitters.

E   Lumpers are more likely than splitters to see similarities.

Questions 9 to 12 refer to the following information:

A school has two rowing teams, Crew A and Crew B. The head coach is considering changing the compositions of the two boats and must calculate the figures for each potential crew's average height and weight.

Crew A position	Height (cm)	Weight (kg)	Crew B position	Height (cm)	Weight (kg)
Seat 1	180	71	Seat 1	167	68
Seat 2	170	65	Seat 2	179	78
Seat 3	180	80	Seat 3	178	70
Seat 4	177	75	Seat 4	169	77
Seat 5	174	69	Seat 5	182	75
Seat 6	182	79	Seat 6	187	76
Seat 7	185	77.5	Seat 7	190	85
Seat 8	172	70.5	Seat 8	193	92
Coxswain	165	56	Coxswain	167	62
Total	1585	643	Total	1612	683

9   Switching which pair of rowers would most affect each crew's average height?

A   Seat 1

B   Seat 2

C   Seat 3

D   Seat 4

E   Seat 5

F   Seat 6

G   Seat 7

H   Seat 8

10   What would be the average weight of Crew B if the coxswains were to be switched (in kgs)?

A   71.4

B   72.1

C   75.2

D   75.9

11   If the coach were to rearrange the crews by putting the heaviest 8 rowers and the heavier coxswain on Crew A and the lightest 8 rowers and the lighter coxswain on Crew B, how many people would have to switch crews?

A   6

B   8

C   10

D   12

12   Which of the following crews does the chart below represent?

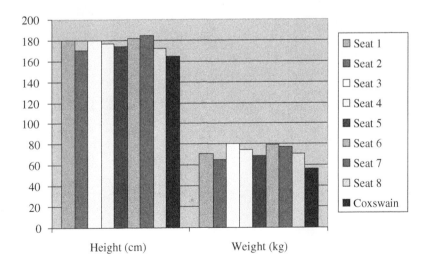

A   The original Crew A

B   The original Crew B

C   Crew A after switching coxswains

D   Crew B after switching coxswains

13 Belton has increased its funding for the arts by 50%, and now its budget for the arts surpasses Allenton's budget for the arts by 50%. But Allenton is renowned for its live theatre, and Belton has no professional theatre troupe. Therefore, the increased funding for the arts in Belton has been ineffective because Allenton is more cultured than Belton.

Which **one** of the following is an underlying assumption of the above argument?

A   Funding for the arts only includes funding for the performing arts.

B   A town's level of culture is determined by a combination of factors, including history, architecture, visual arts and performing arts.

C   Allocations of funds for the arts should be determined on a regional rather than local level.

D   Live theatre is the primary factor in determining whether a city is cultured.

E   The more a city spends on the arts, the more cultured it is.

14   Bianca painted a room 60% pink and 40% cornflower.

Before she started, she had three full 3 litre pots of paint: one red, one blue and one white. She mixed equal parts red and white to create the pink paint and she mixed blue and white in a certain ratio to create the cornflower paint.

Unfortunately, Bianca forgot to write down the ratio used to mix the cornflower paint. However, she notes that she mixed the exact amounts of pink and cornflower paint that she needed. After mixing the paints, Bianca had 600 ml of blue paint and 750 ml of red paint left.

How much white paint did Bianca have left?

A   150 ml

B   175 ml

C   220 ml

D   270 ml

E   285 ml

F   310 ml

15   When the marine police send out patrols to tightly enforce maritime speed limits, the vast majority of boating accidents are prevented. Recently, however, budgetary constraints have compelled the marine police to cut back on speed limit enforcement, which means there will be a sharp increase in the number of boating accidents this year – accidents which could have been prevented.

Why is the reasoning above not logically sound?

A   It ignores the possibility that the marine police may have reallocated its resources to increase public safety.

B   It introduces irrelevant information as evidence in support of its conclusion.

C   It treats something that can cause a certain result as though it were necessary for that result.

D   It disregards the role of other factors such as alcohol consumption in boating accidents.

E   It assumes that boaters will drive recklessly unless there is tight enforcement by marine police.

16   At Debenham Market, the cost of 34 apples and 21 pears is equal to the cost of 16 apples and 33 pears. What percent of the cost of an apple is the cost of a pear at Debenham Market ?

A   25%

B $66\frac{2}{3}\%$

C   75%

D $133\frac{1}{3}\%$

E   150%

17   The mathematics department at St. Mary's School has noted a steady improvement over the years in the quality of work done by its students on both examinations and homework assignment. This shows that, contrary to popular belief, secondary school students are better at mathematics than they used to be.

Which **one** of the following is the most serious flaw in the above argument?

A   It does not distinguish between examination results and the quality of work done on homework.

B   It does not account for the possibility that St. Mary's mathematics teachers are very talented.

C   It mentions but does not adequately address the issue of 'popular belief'.

D   It fails to acknowledge the existence of contrary evidence that might weaken the argument.

E   It offers no proof that the students at St. Mary's School are representative of all secondary school students.

18 A recent athletics meeting included a total of 16 competitors in the Javelin Throw event. In the preliminary round, each competitor was allowed two attempts, with the higher distance counting as their score. The top five scores from the preliminary round, along with anyone within 50 cm of fifth place, went through to the final round later in the meeting.

The distances thrown in the preliminary round are listed in the table.

Competitor number	First throw (m)	Second throw (m)
1	34.69	37.05
2	38.36	36.29
3	37.81	38.74
4	40.58	40.13
5	38.12	42.97
6	37.43	38.47
7	36.67	38.53
8	41.19	37.48
9	36.54	37.61
10	38.51	37.32
11	39.02	37.86
12	38.61	38.07
13	37.92	41.36
14	36.18	36.82
15	36.55	38.90
16	38.29	37.51

How many competitors qualified for the Javelin Throw final?

A   7

B   8

C   9

D   10

E   11

F   12

Questions 19 to 22 are based on the following information:

A survey of recent secondary school and university graduates asked in what field, if any, the graduates were currently employed. The results of the survey appear in the chart below.

Employment Sector	Secondary School Grads	University Grads
Accounting / Finance	2	147
Admin / Office	94	82
Business / Sales	162	150
Education	12	53
Legal	34	22
Medical / Health	57	23
Service	97	61
Other	42	62
Total	**500**	**600**

19   Which of the following most accurately reflects the percentage of secondary school graduates are employed in the fourth most popular field for this group?

A   9%

B   10%

C   11%

D   12%

E   13%

20   Which of the following employment sectors does the pie chart below depict?

Education Level of Employees

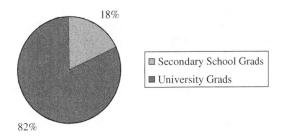

A   Accounting / Finance

B   Admin / Office

C   Business / Sales

D   Education

E   Legal

F   Medical / Health

G   Service

H   Other

21   Which of the following conclusions is justified by the data?

    A   Most university graduates are employed in the Accounting/Finance or Business/Sales sectors.

    B   Within any sector surveyed, non-university graduates make up the greatest percentage of employees surveyed in the Business/Sales sector.

    C   Secondary school grads are more likely to work in the Legal sector than the Service sector.

    D   Most secondary school grads are employed in non-managerial roles.

    E   University graduates are employed at a lower rate than secondary school grads in the Legal sector.

22   Including both secondary school grads and university grads, approximately what percentage of those surveyed are employed in the category labelled as Other?

    A   20.8%

    B   17.3%

    C   9.5%

    D   5.2%

23   There has been a move to eliminate single-use plastics, such as bottles, food containers and disposable cutlery, due to the amount of waste they generate. Whilst many of these single-use plastics can be recycled, in fact they often end up in the oceans, and they account for one-third of all plastic produced in 2017. Thus, a significant reduction in single-use plastics would seriously reduce worldwide plastic production. However, the consequences of a big reduction in single-use plastics will be worse for the environment. The alternative products – such as glass bottles or disposable cutlery made of wood – use up more natural resources and energy. For example, a glass bottle requires 80% more energy to produce than a plastic bottle, with much higher shipping costs – requiring more fuel – due to glass weighing more than plastic.

Which one of the following is an assumption underlying the above argument?

    A   People do not recycle single-use plastics in sufficient quantities.

    B   There are no alternatives to single-use plastics that would not be worse for the environment.

    C   The cost of producing and shipping glass bottles is higher than for plastic bottles.

    D   Reducing our reliance on single-use plastics would drastically cut worldwide plastic production.

24   My bank account number consists of eight digits. None of the digits are repeated.

The sixth digit is 3.

If you break the account number into two 4-digit numbers, these two numbers add up to 10,001.

If you break the first six digits of the account number into two 3-digit numbers, these two numbers add up to 811.

What is the last digit of my passcode?

A   1

B   2

C   4

D   5

E   6

F   7

G   8

H   9

25   For the past twenty years, researchers have used underwater hydrophones to record the vocalisations of blue, fin and humpback whales. The original intent of the study was to see if 'acoustic smog' was affecting whale communication. Acoustic smog is another term for noise pollution, which is increasing as our oceans become more populous. A few years into their work, the researchers discovered that there is a commercial market for the recordings. Whilst their decision to release an album has been criticised in some quarters, it is unfair to attack the researchers for 'selling out' when in fact they have been creative in getting their message out. The haunting, almost melancholy songs of the humpback whale cannot fail to move listeners and raise public awareness of the acoustic threat to whale communication.

Which one of the following, if true, most strengthens the above argument?

A   The researchers believe that noise pollution is a threat to whale communication.

B   Whale watching tours have become more popular because of the recordings, leading to a rise in noise pollution near humpback whales.

C   Whales kept in solitary tanks in sea life parks do not sing.

D   The researchers do not make a profit from the sales of the whale recordings.

E   Funds from each download of the whale album are invested in whale breeding programmes, designed to increase whale populations in the oceans.

26   A jogger consumes a sports drink while running. The graph below marks the runner's intake of calories from the sports drink and expenditure of calories from running during a ten-minute workout.

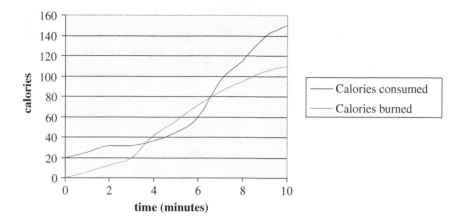

Which one of the following must be true?

A   For the majority of the run, the jogger has consumed enough calories to fuel his workout.

B   The jogger consumes the sports drink at a steady rate whilst running.

C   The rate at which the jogger burns calories increases during the second half of his run.

D   The overall rate at which the jogger consumes calories is lower than the overall rate at which he expends calories.

27   Two couples, Karl and Linda, and Mickey and Nora, attend a fundraising luncheon. Linda is the first to arrive, and sits in a seat facing the stage. Next, Nora arrives, and sits so that she faces neither the stage nor Linda. Mickey arrives, complaining of a sore neck. He asks to sit in the seat facing the stage. Linda moves over one seat, giving Mickey the seat he wants. Karl comes last, and sits in the only seat left, but then switches with Nora.

1.   **Stage**   2.   **Stage**   3.   **Stage**

            Nora   Karl   Mickey

Karl   Linda   Nora   Linda   Karl   Linda

        Mickey   Mickey   Nora

Which of the following could be an accurate representation of the final seating arrangement?

A   1 and 3 only

B   1 and 2 only

C   1 only

D   2 and 3 only

E   3 only

28   A local theatre is putting on a children's musical called Wonderfully Wendy with 8 characters that will be performed by fewer than 8 actors. Wendy, Dawn and Chloe are characters who must be performed by female actors and Ned, Rufus and Elliott must be performed by male actors. There are two adult characters who can be performed by male or female actors. Each actor can perform more than one character but each character can only be performed by one actor. The actor who performs the role of Wendy cannot perform any other characters. The table indicates the characters that appear together in each scene:

scene	characters
1	Wendy and Rufus
2	Wendy, Elliott and Chloe
3	Ned and Chloe
4	Rufus, Elliott and Dawn
5	Wendy, Ned and Adult 2
6	Wendy, Elliott and Adult 1
7	Ned and Dawn
8	Dawn and Chloe
9	Wendy, Rufus and Chloe
10	Ned and Dawn
11	Wendy, Rufus, Elliott and Chloe
12	Rufus, Elliott, Adult 1 and Adult 2

In this production, the actor who performs the role of Chloe also performs the role of Adult 2.

Which of the following pairs of characters could be performed by the same actor in this production?

A   Wendy and Dawn

B   Elliott and Adult 1

C   Dawn and Adult 2

D   Rufus and Ned

E   Dawn and Rufus

F   Chloe and Adult 1

29   A fair die, with sides numbered 1, 2, 3, 4, 5 and 6, is to be rolled 4 times. What is the probability that on at least one roll, the number showing is a 5 or a 6?

   A $\dfrac{8}{81}$

   B $\dfrac{16}{81}$

   C $\dfrac{48}{81}$

   D $\dfrac{65}{81}$

   E $\dfrac{80}{81}$

30   A recent study conducted by a university documents a sharp decline in the amount of time that students spend working in university libraries. The same study shows a sharp increase in the number of students who have their own laptop computers. University administrators have concluded that students are using the libraries less because they are now able to do much of their reading and research online.

   Which **one** of the following, if true, would be a reason to distrust the argument above?

   A   Students with laptop computers are more likely to study in the library than students without laptop computers.

   B   Students without laptop computers are able to read and do research on library computers.

   C   Some students lie in response to questions about their study habits and/or computer use.

   D   Many students believe that online research is easier to do but less accurate than research done in a library.

   E   Many students with laptop computers take them to the library.

31   The figure below is for forming a code. A code is to be formed by placing one of the letters A, B, C or D in space 1, and one of the integers 1, 4, 5, 7 or 8 in each of spaces 2, 3 and 4. How many different codes are possible?

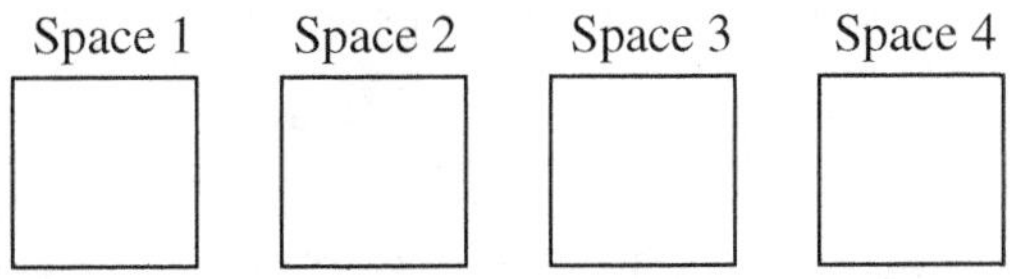

Space 1	Space 2	Space 3	Space 4

A   256

B   320

C   400

D   500

E   625

Questions 32 to 35 refer to the following information:

There are 10,500 fewer pubs in the UK in 2016 than in the year 2000, a decline of 17%. The amount of beer sold in pubs, clubs and restaurants in the UK has fallen by 46% since 2000, whilst the amount of beer sold in UK supermarkets and off-licences has risen by 27% in the same period, surpassing beer sales in pubs, clubs and restaurants for every year since 2014.

The drinking habits of British adults have also changed in the last two decades. In 2005, 65% of British adults reported drinking alcohol the previous week, but this figure dropped to 57% in 2016; 2% of all British adults switched from drinking alcohol the previous week in 2005 to never drinking alcohol in 2016. Some 10.6 million British adults, or 16.1% of the adult population of the UK in 2016, never drink alcohol.

What changed in Britain to affect the number of pubs and adults who drink alcohol since the start of the century? It is commonly believed that the smoking ban is directly responsible for the decline in the number of pubs. Smoking was banned in all enclosed work places in England from 1st July 2007, having been banned in other parts of the UK in the previous 18 months.

The smoking ban was certainly effective. Councils in England inspected 590,155 premises, including pubs, bars, restaurants, clubs and hotels, in the first 18 months following the introduction of the smoking ban on 1st July 2007. 98.2% of these premises were compliant with the smoking ban and 89.3% of these premises displayed the correct 'No smoking' signs. Thus, it seems reasonably likely that the smoking ban discouraged smokers from drinking in pubs and other venues, which could account for the pub closures.

However, there are two problems with this theory. First, it does not account in the shifting figures in alcohol sales and the rise in teetotal Brits (those who never drink alcohol); if smokers stopped drinking in pubs after the smoking ban, one might expect they would account for a parallel rise in alcohol sales in supermarkets and off-licences, but the figures do not bear this out. Second, the effects of the smoking ban may have amplified a long-term decline in smoking in the UK. In 2000, 26.8% of British adults were smokers, but this figure dropped to 19.8% in 2011 and 14.9% in 2017. Specific data for male and female adult smokers in the UK in the last few decades are given in the table below.

Adults aged 16 and over in the UK that smoke						
2000	2006	2007	2011	2012	2016	2017
26%	22%	21%	19.8%	20%	15.5%	14.9%

Prevalence of smoking by sex in the UK, adults aged 16 and over					
Sex	1977	1987	1997	2007	2017
Males	47%	34%	30%	22%	17%
Females	38%	31%	26%	20%	13%

32   To the nearest hundred, how many pubs were there in the UK in the year 2000?

     A   55,600

     B   58,900

     C   61,800

     D   64,700

33   What is the proportion of premises in England inspected by councils from 1st July 2007 to 31st December 2008 that failed to comply with the smoking ban to premises that displayed the correct 'No smoking' signs?

     A   1 in 60

     B   1 in 50

     C   1 in 45

     D   1 in 40

34   Which of the following is supported by the information given?

     1   Smoking was legally permitted in pubs in all parts of the UK in 2005.

     2   The number of adult male smokers in the UK decreased by half from 1987 to 2017.

     A   1 only

     B   2 only

     C   both 1 and 2

     D   neither 1 nor 2

35   If the UK had 26.4 million male adults aged 16 and over in 2017 and 700,000 more female adults in the same age group in the same year, how many more males than females in that age group smoked?

     A   388,000

     B   617,000

     C   844,000

     D   965,000

BMAT SECTION 2: SCIENTIFIC KNOWLEDGE AND APPLICATIONS (30 MINUTES)

You have 30 minutes to answer 27 questions. There are no penalties for incorrect answers, so you should attempt all questions.

Fill in your answers to each question on the answer sheet provided. Shade the circles corresponding to the answer choice(s) you have selected.

Avoid making stray marks on the paper. If you make a mistake, erase your answer completely and try again.

Calculators are **not** permitted.

1   Which graph represents the relationship between current and voltage in a series circuit of constant resistance?

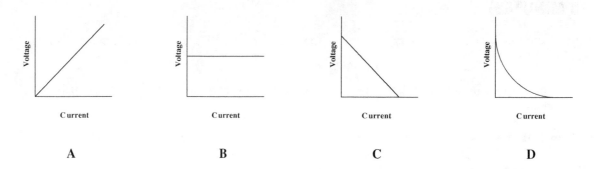

A   B   C   D

2   The entry for calcium in the periodic table is copied below.

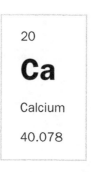

How many neutrons and charged particles are present in a $^{40}Ca^{2+}$ ion?

	neutrons:	charged particles:
A	18	20
B	20	38
C	20	40
D	40	18
E	40	22

3 Which of the following is equal to $\dfrac{5.285 \times 10^{24} + 3.159 \times 10^{28}}{1.057 \times 10^{30}}$?

A 0.0030005

B 0.030005

C 0.30005

D 0.050003

4 A student performs some tests on some unidentified hydrocarbon compounds.

compound	appearance	shake with bromine water	combustion in air
(i)	volatile liquid	orange colour	burns with blue flame
(ii)	light oil	decolourised	burns with yellow flame
(iii)	viscous oil	decolourised	burns with sooty flame
(iv)	viscous oil	orange colour	burns with yellow flame

Which of the following can be determined from these data? Select all that apply.

1 Compound (i) has a lower boiling point than compound (ii).

2 Compound (ii) is an alkene.

3 Compound (iii) is unsaturated.

4 Compounds (i) and (iv) are saturated.

5 Compound (iv) has a higher molecular weight than compound (iii).

A 1, 2 and 4

B 1, 2 and 5

C 1, 3 and 4

D 1, 3 and 5

E 2, 3 and 4

F 2, 4 and 5

G 3, 4 and 5

5   The diagram below is a simple sketch of a nephron, the functional unit of the excretory system. In which of labelled parts of the diagram are the following statements appropriate?

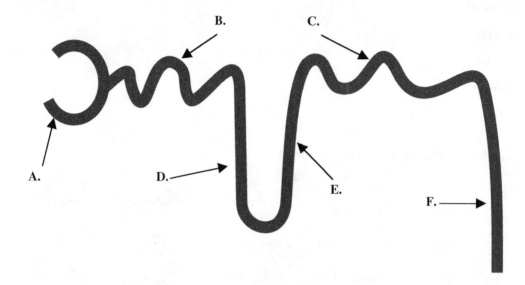

(i)   water is reabsorbed under the control of ADH
(ii)   virtually all amino acids are reabsorbed
(iii) membranes prevent the filtration of proteins
(iv)   active transport of salts takes place into the renal medulla

	(i)	(ii)	(iii)	(iv)
A	F	B	A	E
B	C	D	B	A
C	B	C	A	D
D	D	A	C	E
E	A	F	E	B

6   An electric light is 40% efficient. If 500 Kwatt of electrical power is supplied to the light bulb for 10 seconds, how many joules of light energy will be released?

A   2,000

B   5,000

C   2,000,000

D   5,000,000

7 Which of the following is a correct representation of $y = \dfrac{5x + 30}{6} - \dfrac{3x - 4}{5} - 3$?

A

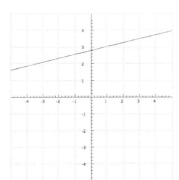

B

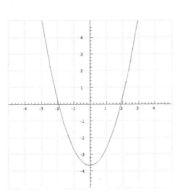

C

D

E

8   The graph shows the activity of an enzyme according to pH.

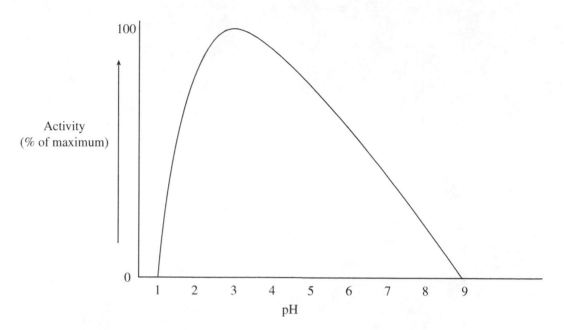

Which of the following statements about this enzyme is true?

A   A mutation in the DNA of the enzyme could result in a change in the shape of the curve.

B   It has an optimum pH of around 2.

C   It could be salivary amylase.

D   The drop to an activity of 0 at a pH of 9 occurs due to the denaturing of the carbohydrate structure of the enzyme.

9   Which of the following would increase the final yield of CO_2 in the following reaction:

$C_6H_{12}O_6 + 6O_2 \rightarrow 6CO_2 + 6H_2O$

A   Increase the amount of H_2O

B   Decrease the amount of O_2

C   Increase the amount of $C_6H_{12}O_6$

D   None of the above

10   Consider the following graph.

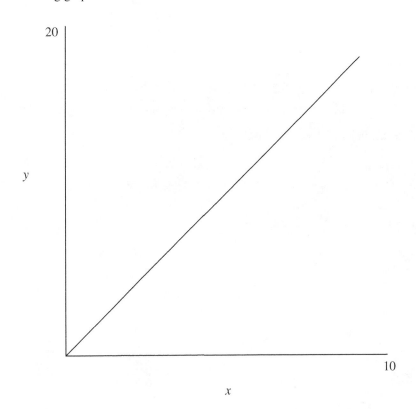

Which row of the table does NOT show a valid combination of the variables x and y, with a correct corresponding interpretation of the gradient of the line?

	x	y	*interpretation of gradient*
A	time (s)	speed (m/s)	an acceleration of 2 m/s^2
B	resistance (Ω)	voltage (V)	a current of 2A
C	weight (N)	mass (kg)	a gravitational field strength of 2 N/kg
D	mass (kg)	resultant force (N)	an acceleration of 2 m/s^2

11   What is the next logical number in the following sequence?

$$0, \quad 1, \quad 3, \quad 7, \quad 15, \quad \underline{\quad}$$

A   17

B   19

C   24

D   31

12   Concerning catalysts, which of the following statements is correct?

    A   Catalysts improve the atom economy of a reaction.

    B   Catalysts increase the reaction enthalpy change.

    C   Catalysts improve the yield of a reaction.

    D   Catalysts reduce the energy costs of industrial processes.

    E   Catalysts act in a different phase to the reaction substrates.

13   If $\sqrt{\dfrac{8}{a} + 8b^2 + 46b + 60} = 3b + 10$, which of the following describes a in terms of b ?

    A $a = \dfrac{(3b+10)^2}{8}$

    B $a = \dfrac{8}{(3b+10)^2}$

    C $a = \dfrac{8}{(b+4)(b+10)}$

    D $a = \dfrac{8}{b^2 + 40}$

14   The following represent anatomical structures in and around the heart:

A	Aortic Arch	**G**	Descending Aorta
B	Superior Vena Cava	**H**	Left Ventricle
C	Right Atrium	**I**	Left Atrium
D	Atrioventricular Valve	**J**	Left Pulmonary Veins
E	Right Ventricle	**K**	Left Pulmonary Arteries
F	Inferior Vena Cava		

Which one of the following represents a path that might be taken by blood passing through a normal adult heart?

    A   C – F – G – J

    B   K – J – I – H

    C   A – B – C – F

    D   H – G – C – F

    E   J – I – C – F

15   A uniform and constant magnetic field is directed into the plane of the page within the square area as shown
      below. A circular loop of wire is moving at constant speed to the right.

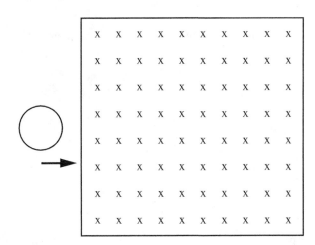

Which of the following graphs best illustrates the induced current in the loop of wire as a function of time?

A
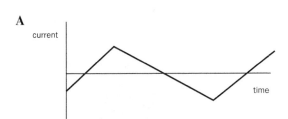

C
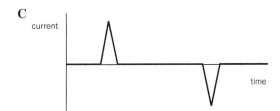

B
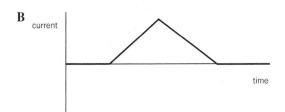

D
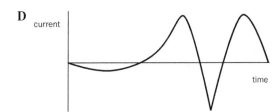

16   The Haber Process of making ammonia is an equilibrium reaction.
        The reaction is exothermic reaction and equation is as follows:

$$N_{2\,(g)} + 3H_{2\,(g)} \leftrightarrow 2NH_{3\,(g)}$$

Given these conditions, which of the following would NOT yield the maximum amount of ammonia?

A   Increasing the pressure

B   Increasing the temperature

C   Increasing the concentration of N_2

D   Decreasing the concentration of NH_3

17   A reflex arc allows an automatic response to a stimulus without the need for a decision by the brain.

Which answer choice lists in the correct order the following events that occur during the activity of a reflex arc?

(i)   transmission to CNS
(ii)   activation of effector
(iii)   transmission by relay neurone
(iv)   transmission by motor neurone
(v)   activation of peripheral receptor

A   (iv) → (v)   → (ii)   → (i)   → (iii)

B   (ii) → (v)   → (iii) → (i)   → (iv)

C   (v)   → (iii) → (i)   → (iv)   → (ii)

D   (i)   → (v)   → (iii) → (ii)   → (iv)

E   (v)   → (i)   → (iii) → (iv)   → (ii)

18   Two long wires 1 and 2 separated by a distance d conduct current in opposite directions.

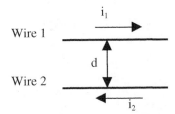

Which of the following statements is true?

A   The magnetic field created by i_2 creates a net force on wire 1 only.

B   The magnetic field created by i_2 creates a net force on both wires.

C   The magnetic field created by i_2 creates a net force on wire 2 only.

D   The magnetic field created by i_2 does not create a net force on either wire.

19 The diagram shows a conical flask containing 0.02 mol hydrochloric acid. A bung connected to a gas syringe is attached to the flask, and the volume of gas initially in the syringe is shown.

An excess of calcium is added to the flask and the bung immediately replaced. The reaction produces hydrogen gas and calcium chloride.

What is the final volume of gas in the syringe?

(1 mol of gas occupies 24 dm^3 at RTP)

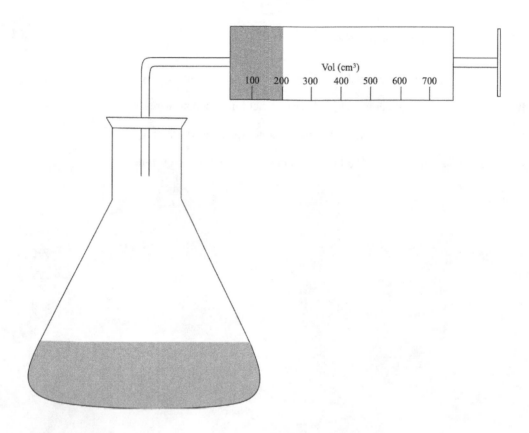

A 240 cm^3

B 440 cm^3

C 480 cm^3

D 680 cm^3

20   Inhalation begins with the onset of contraction of the diaphragm, which results in:

	volume of thoracic cavity	intrathoracic pressure	airflow direction	blood flow to heart
A	decreases	increases	from bronchi to trachea	increases
B	decreases	decreases	from trachea to bronchi	no change
C	increases	decreases	from trachea to bronchi	decreases
D	increases	increases	from bronchi to trachea	no change
E	increases	decreases	from trachea to bronchi	increases

21   A 10 kg, 100 kg, and a 1,000 kg mass are placed on a frictionless inclined plane with a height 10 m. All three masses are released at the same time and the final velocities of the three masses are recorded. How will the final velocity of the three masses compare?

A   The 10 kg mass will have the highest final velocity.

B   The 100 kg mass will have the highest final velocity.

C   The 1,000 kg mass will have the highest final velocity.

D   All three masses will have the same final velocity.

22   The combustion of ethane results in carbon dioxide and water. The equation for this reaction is:

$$w\, C_2H_6 + x\, O_2 \rightarrow y\, CO_2 + z\, H_2O$$

What is the value of x?

A   2

B   3

C   4

D   5

E   6

F   7

23   In the diagram, O is the centre of the circle, the length of WX is $3\sqrt{3}$, and the area of the circle is 36π. What is the area of the shaded region?

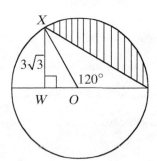

A $12\pi - 18\sqrt{3}$ B $12\pi - 9\sqrt{3}$ C $12\pi - \dfrac{9\sqrt{3}}{2}$ D $36\pi - 9\sqrt{3}$

Questions 24 and 25 refer to the following information:

After eating, glucose from food is released into the blood stream. In response, insulin is produced by specialised cells in the pancreas called β cells. This insulin binds to insulin receptors on the surface of cells throughout the body and signals cells to take up glucose from the blood stream so that it may be used to produce energy. Certain people have deficiencies in this insulin pathway, which results in diabetes. Diabetics, if untreated, maintain inappropriately high blood sugars.

24   Which of the following is unlikely to be a mechanism of diabetes?

  A   An inability to produce insulin.

  B   A resistance to insulin receptor signalling.

  C   An autoimmune destruction of β cells.

  D   An increased binding of insulin to insulin receptors.

25   Which of the following is unlikely to be an effective way to treat diabetes?

  A   Use medicines to increase insulin sensitivity.

  B   Provide exogenous insulin.

  C   Use medicines that bind to insulin and block binding to the insulin receptor.

  D   Use medicines to decrease sugar absorption in the gastrointestinal system.

26   In the diagram below, BD is parallel to AE, the length of BC is y, and the length of CD is 3y − 10.

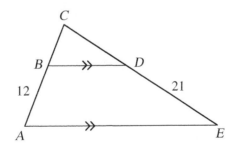

What is the value of y ?

  A   3

  B   4

  C   6

  D   8

27 A circuit is arranged as shown.

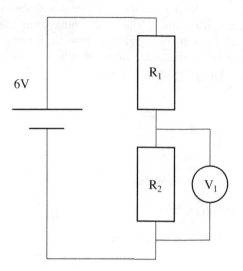

6V

R$_1$

R$_2$ V$_1$

Which of the following could be correct values for R$_1$, R$_2$ and V$_1$?

	R$_1$/Ω	R$_2$/Ω	V$_1$/V
A	10	12	3
B	6	12	4
C	9	10	3
D	5	8	4
E	12	10	3

BMAT SECTION 3: WRITING TASK (30 MINUTES)

Section 3 contains a choice of three tasks. You have 30 minutes in which to answer **one**. You can take notes and make an outline in the space provided in the test booklet, but your answer must be written within the space provided on the answer sheet.

There is no correct answer to any of the questions posed. The writing task provides you with an opportunity to demonstrate your ability to:

- organise and develop your thoughts, and
- produce clear and concise written communication

Be sure to take time to organise your ideas and develop an outline. You may not use a dictionary but you may include a drawing or diagram.

Remember that you have only 30 minutes to select your task, organise your thoughts, and complete your essay.

USE THIS SPACE FOR NOTES

Answer <u>one</u> of the following questions.

1   **If it can't be expressed in figures, it is not science; it is opinion.**

(Lazarus Long)

What does the author mean by this statement? Can you define science in a way that does not limit it to data? What criteria would you use to define whether a hypothesis or theory constitutes 'science'?

2   **Nothing is more fatal to health than over care of it.**

(Benjamin Franklin)

Write an essay in which you address the following points:

What constitutes 'over care' of health, and how can it be 'fatal'? What are the dangers in trying to 'minimise' care? How can doctors take a balanced approach?

3   **Be careful about reading health books. You may die of a misprint.**

(Mark Twain)

What problems can arise when patients try to diagnose and treat themselves? On the other hand, how can popular publications contribute to good health? How can a doctor help a patient who thinks he is well-informed, but isn't?

BMAT TEST 3 – ANSWER KEY

SECTION 1	
Question	Answer
1	C
2	C
3	F
4	B
5	E
6	D
7	E
8	A
9	H
10	C
11	D
12	A
13	D
14	A
15	C
16	E
17	E
18	C
19	C
20	D
21	E
22	C
23	B
24	H
25	A
26	A
27	A
28	D
29	D
30	A
31	D
32	C
33	B
34	A
35	D

SECTION 2	
Question	Answer
1	A
2	B
3	B
4	C
5	A
6	C
7	B
8	A
9	D
10	C
11	C
12	D
13	C
14	B
15	C
16	B
17	E
18	A
19	B
20	E
21	D
22	F
23	B
24	D
25	C
26	D
27	B

BMAT TEST 3 – SCORING TABLES

1. Count up your number of correct answers in each section. Each question is worth one mark.
2. Write the total number of marks correct in each section on the lines below.
3. Find your approximate score for each section in the table below.

	NUMBER CORRECT	APPROXIMATE BMAT SCORE
Section 1	_____	_____
Section 2	_____	_____

SECTION 1		SECTION 2	
Number Correct	BMAT Score	Number Correct	BMAT Score
0	1.0	0	1.0
1	1.0	1	1.0
2	1.0	2	1.0
3	1.0	3	1.3
4	1.0	4	1.8
5	1.1	5	2.2
6	1.5	6	2.6
7	1.9	7	2.9
8	2.2	8	3.2
9	2.5	9	3.5
10	2.8	10	3.7
11	3.1	11	4.0
12	3.4	12	4.2
13	3.6	13	4.5
14	3.9	14	4.7
15	4.1	15	4.9
16	4.4	16	5.2
17	4.6	17	5.4
18	4.9	18	5.6
19	5.1	19	5.9
20	5.4	20	6.2
21	5.6	21	6.5
22	5.9	22	6.8
23	6.1	23	7.2
24	6.4	24	7.7
25	6.7	25	8.3
26	7.0	26	9.0
27	7.3	27	9.0
28	7.6		
29	8.0		
30	8.4		
31	8.9		
32	9.0		
33	9.0		
34	9.0		
35	9.0		

N.B. These scores are for approximation purposes only. The scoring tables used for the BMAT vary slightly year to year, depending on student performance and the norming of the questions in each version of the test paper. To err on the side of caution, these scoring tables are among the toughest ever used on the BMAT. In most cases, a similar performance on the BMAT would result in a slightly higher score.

Test 4

BMAT
Section 1

Test ID

Test 1 ○ Test 2 ○ Test 3 ○ Test 4 ● Test 5 ○

Last Name

First Name

Date

Completely fill in the space for your intended answer choice

A B C D E
○ ○ ● ○ ○

1 A B C D E F
○ ○ ○ ○ ○ ○

2 A B C D
○ ○ ○ ○

3 A B C D
○ ○ ○ ○

4 A B C D E
○ ○ ○ ○ ○

5 A B C D E
○ ○ ○ ○ ○

6 A B C D E
○ ○ ○ ○ ○

7 A B C D
○ ○ ○ ○

8 A B C D E
○ ○ ○ ○ ○

9 A B C D
○ ○ ○ ○

10 A B C D
○ ○ ○ ○

11 A B C D
○ ○ ○ ○

12 A B C D
○ ○ ○ ○

13 A B C D
○ ○ ○ ○

14 A B C D E F G H
○ ○ ○ ○ ○ ○ ○ ○

15 A B C D E
○ ○ ○ ○ ○

16 A B C D E F
○ ○ ○ ○ ○ ○

17 A B C D E
○ ○ ○ ○ ○

18 A B C D E
○ ○ ○ ○ ○

19 A B C D E
○ ○ ○ ○ ○

20 A B C D E
○ ○ ○ ○ ○

21 A B C D E
○ ○ ○ ○ ○

22 A B C D
○ ○ ○ ○

23 A B C D E
○ ○ ○ ○ ○

24 A B C D E
○ ○ ○ ○ ○

25 A B C D E
○ ○ ○ ○ ○

26 A B C D
○ ○ ○ ○

27 A B C D E
○ ○ ○ ○ ○

28 A B C D
○ ○ ○ ○

29 A B C D E
○ ○ ○ ○ ○

30 A B C D
○ ○ ○ ○

31 A B C D E
○ ○ ○ ○ ○

32 A B C D
○ ○ ○ ○

33 A B C D
○ ○ ○ ○

34 A B C D
○ ○ ○ ○

35 A B C D E
○ ○ ○ ○ ○

BMAT is a registered trademark of Cambridge Assessment, which neither sponsors nor endorses this product.

K 145

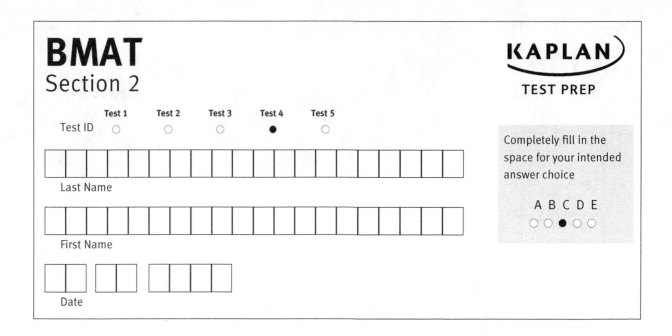

BMAT
Section 2

Test ID Test 1 ○ Test 2 ○ Test 3 ○ Test 4 ● Test 5 ○

Last Name

First Name

Date

1 A B C D
○ ○ ○ ○

2 A B C D E
○ ○ ○ ○ ○

3 A B C D E
○ ○ ○ ○ ○

4 A B C D E
○ ○ ○ ○ ○

5 A B C D E F
○ ○ ○ ○ ○ ○

6 A B C D E
○ ○ ○ ○ ○

7 A B C D E F
○ ○ ○ ○ ○ ○

8 A B C D
○ ○ ○ ○

9 A B C D E F
○ ○ ○ ○ ○ ○

10 A B C D E
○ ○ ○ ○ ○

11 A B C D E
○ ○ ○ ○ ○

12 A B C D
○ ○ ○ ○

13 A B C D E
○ ○ ○ ○ ○

14 A B C D E F G
○ ○ ○ ○ ○ ○ ○

15 A B C D E F
○ ○ ○ ○ ○ ○

16 A B C D E
○ ○ ○ ○ ○

17 A B C D
○ ○ ○ ○

18 A B C D E F
○ ○ ○ ○ ○ ○

19 A B C D E F G
○ ○ ○ ○ ○ ○ ○

20 A B C D E
○ ○ ○ ○ ○

21 A B C D E
○ ○ ○ ○ ○

22 A B C D E F
○ ○ ○ ○ ○ ○

23 A B C D E
○ ○ ○ ○ ○

24 A B C D E F G
○ ○ ○ ○ ○ ○ ○

25 A B C D
○ ○ ○ ○

26 A B C D E
○ ○ ○ ○ ○

27 A B C D
○ ○ ○ ○

BMAT
Section 3

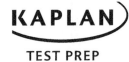

TEST PREP

Last Name

First Name

Question answered ☐

Your answer must be contained within this area.

BMAT is a registered trademark of Cambridge Assessment, which neither sponsors nor endorses this product.

147

BMAT SECTION 1: APTITUDE AND SKILLS (60 MINUTES)

You have 60 minutes to answer 35 questions. There are no penalties for incorrect answers, so you should attempt all questions.

Fill in your answers to each question on the answer sheet provided. Shade the circles corresponding to the answer choice(s) you have selected.

Avoid making stray marks on the paper. If you make a mistake, erase your answer completely and try again.

Calculators are **not** permitted.

1   In a recent survey, people in the UK and around the world were asked to name the most important factor affecting the supply of food. Their responses are shown in the charts below.

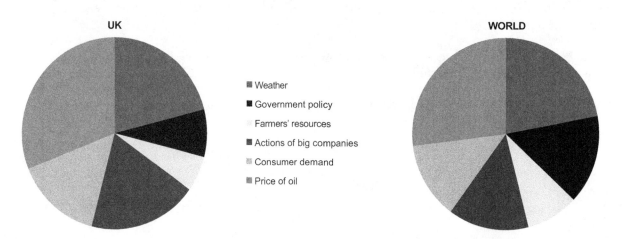

Which of the following statements can be correctly inferred from the data above?

1   People in the UK are more likely than people worldwide to think that the actions of big companies are the most important factor affecting the supply of food.

2   People worldwide are twice as likely as people in the UK to think that farmers' resources are the most important factor affecting the price of food.

3   People worldwide are about twice as likely as people in the UK to think that government policy is the most important factor affecting the food supply.

A   None

B   1 only

C   2 only

D   1 and 2

E   1 and 3

F   All

2   Most metropolitan areas in the country have too many hospitals, and the expenses associated with operating these hospitals are a major drain on the NHS budget. Our cities could get by with far fewer hospitals, and the reduction in facilities and staff salaries could then be spent on GPs, prescription drugs and other services that provide a greater benefit to patients.

Which one of the following, if true, would be most likely to weaken the argument above?

A   Essential medical procedures and tests that are not available in GP surgeries make up the vast majority of operating expenses at metropolitan hospitals.

B   Salaries for specialist doctors and nurses make up the vast majority of operating expenses at metropolitan hospitals.

C   Most patients in metropolitan areas did not visit a hospital as a patient in the last year, but did visit a GP surgery.

D   Most patients in metropolitan areas have taken at least one prescription drug in the last year.

3   I have a standard deck of playing cards, which contains cards of 13 possible values in 4 different suits, for a total of 52 cards. A friend draws a card from the deck at random, and holds on to it. I draw a second card from the deck at random, and hold on to it. My friend then draws a third card from the deck at random. What are the odds that all three cards have the same value?

A $\dfrac{1}{400}$

B $\dfrac{1}{410}$

C $\dfrac{1}{420}$

D $\dfrac{1}{425}$

4   An online farming game gives its users 30 credits each day they log in. One acre of farmland costs 12 credits, and planting one acre of farmland costs 1 credit. Lucy has 5 planted acres and 10 credits in the game before logging in on a Monday, and she proceeds to log in every day that follows, always buying and planting the maximum acreage she can afford with her total credits each day. On what day of the week will Lucy buy and plant her hundredth acre of farmland?

A   Tuesday

B   Wednesday

C   Friday

D   Saturday

E   Sunday

Questions 5 and 6 refer to the following argument.

New Government guidelines recommend that adults eat no more than 500 g of red meat or processed meat per week, or an average of about 70 g per day, to reduce the risk of bowel cancer. The new daily limit is equal to two slices of roast beef or three slices of ham. Popular meals, such as spaghetti bolognese, doner kebab and full English breakfasts are not advisable under the new guidelines; each of these delicious and very popular meals includes twice the daily limit of red meat.

5   Which one of the following best summarises the conclusion of the argument above?

    A   People can limit their chances of developing bowel cancer by limiting how much red meat they eat.

    B   The Government recommends that people should not eat as much meat as they currently do.

    C   Adults can limit their chances of developing bowel cancer by limiting how much red meat they eat.

    D   Eating too much meat can cause bowel cancer.

    E   Eating popular meals can cause cancer.

6   Which one of the following can be most properly inferred from the argument above?

    A   Adults who do not eat a full English breakfast every day are less likely to develop bowel cancer than those who do.

    B   Adults who eat spaghetti bolognese every day are more likely to develop bowel cancer than those who do not eat red meat.

    C   Adults who do not eat ham every day are less likely to develop bowel cancer than those who do.

    D   Vegetarians are less likely to develop bowel cancer than are people who eat red meat.

    E   People who eat a doner kebab three times a week are less likely to develop bowel cancer than those who do not.

7   A large, L-shaped section of floor is to be laid with small L-shaped tiling units. Each tiling unit consists of four squares that are each one foot by one foot, in the shape shown below. Each tiling unit is double-sides, so it can be rotated and flipped into any flat position. All tiling units must be fitted perfectly, so there is no portion of the L-shaped section of floor not covered by tiling units. Which of the following CANNOT be the total surface area of the L-shaped section of floor?

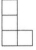

A   16 sq ft

B   40 sq ft

C   48 sq ft

D   62 sq ft

8   The graph below plots the cumulative lengths of terms in office of British prime ministers from 1721 to the present. The y-axis indicates the number of prime ministers who had served no longer than the number of years on the x-axis.

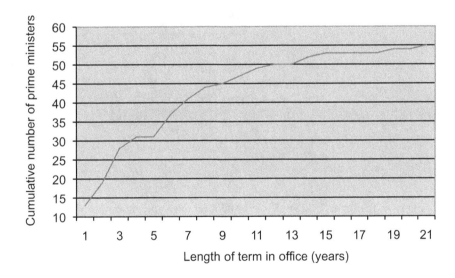

How many prime ministers served for at least 9 years, but no longer than 19 years?

A   7

B   9

C   11

D   45

E   49

Questions 9 to 12 refer to the following information.

The table below gives the expenditures for the Department of Communities and Local Government for 2010.

Category	Expenditure
Communities	£109,451,163
Finance	£457,406,444
Housing	£1,852,774,942
Human Resources	£1,306,360
Local Government	£17,319,826,075
Regions	£203,277,540
Other	£66,544
Total	£19,944,109,068

Spending in most government departments was cut significantly from 2009 levels in 2010, due to a change in government and a newfound emphasis on reducing spending. Financial experts estimated that the cuts to the Department of Communities and Local Government budget would result in an average cut of 10 per cent across all of the UK's local authorities in the next year, though the government spokesman claimed that the average cut to local authorities would be only 4.4%, when all projected revenue streams are taken fully into account.

9   Expenditures on local government represent what percentage of the department's total expenditures?

A   80%

B   83%

C   87%

D   90%

10   28% of expenditures in the 'Other' category were spent on the Strategic Future Unit. How much was spent on the Strategic Future Unit?

A   £17,937

B   £18,646

C   £19,301

D   £19,952

11   In 2009, under the previous government, the department had planned for a series of special projects, bringing its total budget to £36,364,731,000. What is the percentage decrease in the total budget, from 2009 to 2010?

A   37%

B   40%

C   42%

D   45%

12   Which one of the following, if true, would be most likely to weaken the government spokesman's claim that budget cuts will result in a lower average cut to local authority spending than estimated by financial experts?

A   Government projections for local authority revenue streams assume that council tax rates will be frozen at current levels or will rise at a rate below the rate of inflation, but virtually all local authorities have budgeted a rise in council tax rates above the rate of inflation.

B   Government projections for local authority revenue streams assume that council tax rates will rise next year at a rate equal to or above the rate of inflation, but virtually all local authorities have frozen council tax rates at current levels or budgeted a rise below the rate of inflation.

C   All the financial experts whose estimate differed from that of the government spokesman are members of the party that was defeated in the 2010 elections.

D   Cuts in expenditures on council housing are reflected entirely in the budget for the Department of Communities and Local Government, but are not projected to impact the revenue streams for local authorities in any other way.

13   An author is considering two options for publishing her new novel.

Option A: E-book sales: Author to receive royalties of 35% on average retail price of £0.99 per book sold.

Option B: Hardcover sales: Author to receive royalties of 5% on average retail price of £11.99 per book sold.

If the novel sells 100,000 copies, how much more will the author earn in royalties with Option B, rather than Option A?

A   £22,750

B   £23,500

C   £25,300

D   £26,250

14   The European Southern Observatory (ESO) is not located in Europe, but rather in the South American country of Chile. The ESO is found in the Atacama Desert among the mountains of northern Chile, where the skies are incredibly clear and rain is an especially rare occurrence; parts of the desert have never recorded rain. The political stability of Chile over the last few decades has made it the preferred country for astronomers wanting to observe the skies in the Southern Hemisphere. For these reasons, European engineers are designing and building a new observatory, the Extremely Large Telescope (ELT) near the ESO in the Andes. When completed, the ELT will be the most powerful telescope in the world, capable of generating images more than 15 times clearer than those captured in outer space by the Hubble telescope, which are currently the clearest and most powerful images of other planets available. This remarkable optical power, concentrating in an Earth-bound observatory, will assist astronomers in observing other planets like nothing before in the history of science, and will provide the best chance so far of finding signs of life elsewhere in the universe.

Which of the following statements can be correctly inferred from the information above?

1   European observatories are not located in Europe.
2   Astronomers prefer to work in climates that are not especially rainy.
3   Chile is the best country for astronomy.
4   No other telescope generates images of other planets more clearly than the Hubble telescope.

A   2 only

B   3 only

C   1 and 2

D   1 and 3

E   2 and 3

F   2 and 4

G   1, 2 and 3

H   2, 3 and 4

Questions 15 and 16 refer to the information below.

A survey by a major insurance company and the National Union of Students has revealed the popularity of expensive gadgets among university students. According to the survey, all university students own a mobile phone; the percentage of these that own smartphones are shown in the graph below. The average student will take gadgets worth £1,165 to university; by comparison, the average student will keep £542 worth of clothing in their university wardrobe.

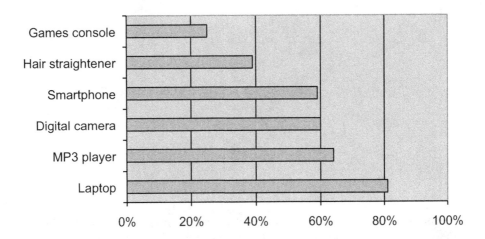

Many students forget to insure their possessions, which can lead to major problems in the unlikely but possible case of theft or fire. Whilst at university, students have two options for insuring their belongings: they can add their valuables to the home insurance taken out by their parents, or they can take out their own policy. Students who opt to join their parents' insurance must be sure to list all valuable items, and also check that their accommodation meets the insurance company's security requirements. For instance, most insurers will require adequate locks on a student's room in a shared house or flat; in a hall of residence, insurers will expect the university to provide a high level of security. Students will still be liable for any excess, but insuring those valuable gadgets has become an essential part of the university experience.

15   According to the information above, which one of the following would be most likely to ensure an entirely successful insurance payout on a claim by a student who has all his gadgets stolen from his university accommodation?

A   The student claims exemption from paying the excess, due to his status as a student.

B   The student claims that his gadgets are covered on his parents' home insurance, but they never filed the paperwork to add his gadgets to their policy.

C   The student claims that his gadgets were stolen from his parents' house, so that they will be covered under his parents' home insurance.

D   The student lives in a hall of residence with extensive CCTV coverage that can be accessed only by scanning a student ID, which is then checked by a security guard who is on duty 24 hours a day, 7 days a week.

E   The student's policy lists his laptop, mobile phone and MP3 player, but not the hair straightener and games console that he received as birthday gifts the day before the theft.

16   Which of the following statements can be correctly inferred from the information?

   1   Some university students own a hair straightener and a digital camera.
   2   Most university students own laptop and an MP3 player.
   3   Most university students own at least two gadgets.
   4   Most university students own smartphones.

   A   1 and 2

   B   1 and 3

   C   2 and 3

   D   1 and 4

   E   2 and 4

   F   3 and 4

17   The last few winters in the UK have proven especially harsh, with several major snowfalls of 5 to 8 inches in 24 hours. Only a few local authorities in the UK have the snow ploughs required to clear roads after such 'blizzards', as gritting salt is only effective with snowfalls of 3 inches or less. Due to the lack of appropriate snow-clearing equipment, thousands of schools have to shut for several days each winter, causing a severe knock-on effect as parents must make expensive, last-minute child-care arrangements, or otherwise stay home from work to watch their children. Even worse was the disruption to UK air travel caused by a blizzard in December 2010. Heathrow had no equipment to clear snow from planes parked at passenger gates, and as a result hundreds of such planes had to be dug out by hand. Severe flight delays followed for the next five days, costing the airlines and the British economy to lose tens of millions of pounds. In order to prevent a repeat of these massive losses and inconveniences, UK airports and local authorities must make significant investment in snow-clearing equipment their top priority before next winter.

Which one of the following is the best statement of the central assumption in the argument above?

   A   Nothing is more important for UK airports and local authorities than preventing loss and inconvenience.

   B   Winters will be especially harsh for the foreseeable future.

   C   Airports should pay any cost required to prevent inconvenience to passengers.

   D   The cost of preventing inconvenience due to snow is not greater than the economic losses due to snow.

   E   Local authorities with appropriate snow-clearing equipment never have to shut schools due to heavy snowfall.

18   An alphanumeric code is based on the numeric value of letters of the alphabet (eg, A = 1, B = 2, C = 3). The code adds a set 'adjustment' to numeric value of each letter, and the adjustment is encoded using a 'keyword' that spells out the value of the adjustment after it has been added to each letter.

EXAMPLE: If the adjustment has a value of 2, then the keyword is VYQ. This adds the adjustment to each letter of TWO:

$$T = 20; 20 + 2 = 22 = V$$
$$W = 23; 23 + 2 = 25 = Y$$
$$O = 15; 15 + 2 = 17 = Q$$

Subtract 26 to find the letter if the adjustment value results in a new value larger than 26; eg with an adjustment of 25, then X becomes W, as X = 24; 24 + 25 = 49; 49 − 26 = 23 = W.

Which of the following is encoded correctly as a keyword, using the alphanumeric code?

A   KNDJ

B   MCR

C   FKQAKK

D   TXTFSST

E   JVMVEKVVE

Question 19 to 22 refer to the following information:

The bar chart below shows the profits of company *X* in the five regions in which the company conducts business. The profits are shown for June and July.

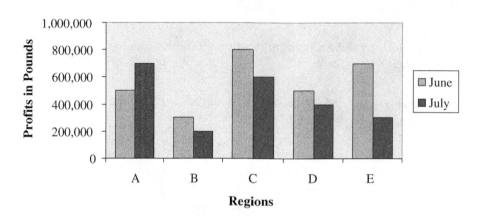

Profits of Company X

19   By approximately what percent did the profits in region D decrease from June to July?

    A   20%

    B   25%

    C $37\frac{1}{2}\%$

    D $62\frac{1}{2}\%$

    E   75%

20   If in August, each of regions A, B, C and D had the same profits that they had in July while the profits in region E were £85,000 less than they were in July, how many pounds less than the average of the profits, in pounds, for the five regions in July would the average of the profits, in pounds, for the five regions in August be?

    A   1,250

    B   15,000

    C   16,000

    D   17,000

    E   20,000

21   The profits of company *X*, in pounds, in the five regions in June is shown correctly in which of the following columns?

	Column 1	Column 2	Column 3	Column 4	Column 5
Region *A*	700,000	500,000	500,000	700,000	700,000
Region *B*	200,000	300,000	300,000	200,000	300,000
Region *C*	600,000	600,000	800,000	800,000	800,000
Region *D*	400,000	400,000	500,000	500,000	400,000
Region *E*	300,000	300,000	700,000	700,000	300,000

A   Column 1

B   Column 2

C   Column 3

D   Column 4

E   Column 5

22   Which of the following pie charts shows the correct proportions of the company's profits in July in the 5 regions?

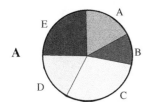

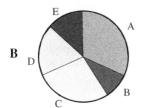

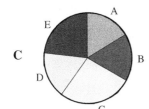

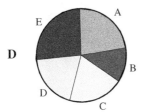

23   A recent study conducted by a university documents a sharp decline in the amount of time that students spend working in university libraries. The same study shows a sharp increase in the number of students who have their own laptop computers. University administrators have concluded that students are using the libraries less because they are now able to do much of their reading and research online.

Which **one** of the following, if true, would be a reason to distrust the argument above?

A   Students with laptop computers are more likely to study in the library than students without laptop computers.

B   Students without laptop computers are able to read and do research on library computers.

C   Some students lie in response to questions about their study habits and/or computer use.

D   Many students believe that online research is easier to do but less accurate than research done in a library.

E   Many students with laptop computers take them to the library.

24   Five friends sit at a round table that has six seats. No one sits directly opposite Gerry. Harold can sit only next to Frida, John or an empty seat. Inga and Gerry sit next to one another.

Which **one** of the following is an acceptable seating arrangement?

A   Empty, Frida, Harold, John, Inga, Gerry

B   Empty, John, Inga, Frida, Gerry, Harold

C   Gerry, Inga, Frida, Empty, John, Harold

D   Gerry, Frida, Harold, Empty, John, Inga

E   Gerry, Empty, Frida, Harold, John, Inga

25   Many people in Australia believe that industry is the biggest contributor to air pollution, but this is not true. The biggest single source is exhaust from automobiles. If the government truly wants to attack the country's air pollution problem, it should stop focusing so much on industry and build up its public transportation system.

Which **one** of the following, if true, strengthens the above argument?

A   Industrial transportation is not a major source of automotive exhaust.

B   The government can afford to improve public transportation.

C   The government wants to attack the country's air pollution problem.

D   Industry will not voluntarily cut profits to improve air quality.

E   People in Australia are willing to make sacrifices to improve air quality.

26   The speeds of different vehicles A, B, C and D are shown during a 5-minute interval. Which vehicle travelled the greatest distance in the 5 minutes?

A

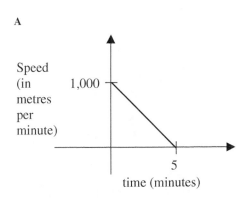

B

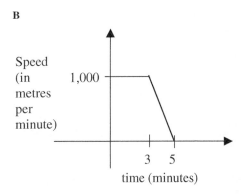

C

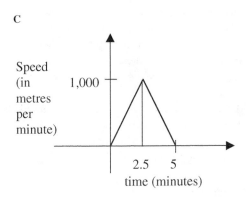

D

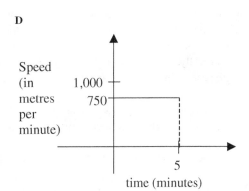

27   Marcus has been called a bad composer, by critics who say he is more interested in experimenting with strange musical notation and new instruments than he is in pleasing his audience. One only has to look, however, at the music of revered composer John Cage to see that this critique is unjustified. Cage was called 'innovative' and 'brilliant' for his use of weird notation and invented instruments.

Which **one** of the following is a flaw in the above argument?

A   It fails to precisely define the term 'interested'.

B   It seeks to undermine the critics on the basis of one counter-example.

C   It assumes that Cage was not interested in pleasing his audience.

D   It assumes that Marcus is as good as Cage.

E   It fails to demonstrate that Cage was a good composer.

28   As part of a Bank Holiday sales promotion, the price of a used car is discounted by 10% each day of the Bank Holiday weekend, from Friday to Monday. By the time the sales promotion ends on Monday, by what total percentage has the price of the car been discounted from its original price on Thursday?

A   60%

B   66%

C   68%

D   73%

29   Consumers should be very careful about switching their electricity provider in response to a salesperson who calls at their home. According to figures released by the energy regulator, some 40% of customers who switched providers in response to doorstep sales tactics ended up paying more for their electricity than they had previously. Generally, there are savings to be had by switching electricity providers, but consumers are likely to realise the greatest savings if they have never switched previously, or if they switch to direct debit from other methods of payment. This is all to say that despite the best efforts of electricity providers to increase sales and generate revenue by encouraging customers to switch providers, at the end of the day consumers are likely to find that little, if any, difference in their tariff results from switching energy companies.

Which one of the following best summarises the main point of the argument above?

A   Most people save money on their electricity by switching energy providers.

B   The energy regulator could do more to stop the deceptive sales practices of some energy companies.

C   You will reduce your electricity tariff by switching your payments to direct debit.

D   You should not believe what energy companies tell you.

E   You are unlikely to save money on your electricity by switching energy providers.

30   Ash subscribes to home broadband with a top download speed of 20Mb per second, and a guaranteed minimum download speed of 2Mb per second. He notes that 1 MB (megabyte) = 8 Mb (megabits). Ash wants to download an episode of his favourite TV programme, with a total file size of 660MB. How much longer will it take for the file to download if it does so entirely at the slowest speed, as compared to entirely at top speed?

A   4 minutes, 24 seconds

B   36 minutes, 48 seconds

C   39 minutes, 36 seconds

D   44 minutes

31   Reliable studies have shown that operator error is a factor in most big wheel accidents. To address this problem, funfairs have improved their operator training programmes by adding an observation period, and a period during which new operators are 'shadowed' and supervised by more experienced operators. It is, however, unrealistic to expect these improvements to adequately compensate for the operators' inexperience. The funfairs should therefore reconsider their approach to reducing accidents.

Which **one** of the following is taken for granted in the above argument?

A   Improved training programmes are the best way to reduce accidents.

B   Lack of experience is a significant factor in operator error.

C   Training programmes cannot address issues such as mechanical failure.

D   Experienced operators make fewer errors than inexperienced operators.

E   Operators go through training more than once in their careers.

Questions 32 to 35 refer to the following information:

In 1855, excavations at the site of the ancient city of Larsa, in present-day Iraq, unearthed a large number of tablets traceable to Sumero-Babylonian times, approximately 1900–1500 B.C. The materials appeared to be receipts, accounts and tables. Interpretation revealed that the number system of this ancient civilisation was sexagesimal (counting was by 10s and 60s).

It is now known that not only the number system but also the system of linear measure used by the Sumero- Babylonian society was based on 60. A clay tablet recovered at Larsa some time after the initial findings, believed to be a standard text copied as part of the school curriculum, shows a system of linear measure utilising units that represented specific quantities of barley, the society's food staple and currency. Six she(grains) were equal to 1 shu-si (finger), 30 shu-si equalled 1 kush (cubit), 12 kush equalled 1 nindan, 60 nindan equalled 1 USH, and 30 USH added up to 1 beru. The factors used to convert from one unit to another – 6, 30, 12, 60, and 30 – are multiples of six, and each is a factor of 60, the base in the sexagesimal number system.

Later excavations revealed that the Sumero-Babylonian mathematical system was a successor of sexagesimal systems that had appeared both in earlier eras and in other geographical locations. Tablet fragments discovered in the 1920s at Jemdet Nasr in Iraq disclosed that the numerical and linear systems first noted in 1855 probably had been in use as early as 2900-2800 B.C. The pictographic inscriptions appeared to be a precursor of a Sumerian form of writing known as cuneiform. The notations reflected computation in multiples of 10 and 60 while the basic unit of measure was the she or grain. The Jemdet Nasr findings are thus considered proto-Sumerian.

Research at Susa, the ancient Elamite city located in present-day Iran, has revealed that this separate culture probably used the mathematical system noted at the Sumerian sites. Initial excavations at Susa uncovered tablets inscribed with both the cuneiform writings and numerals of Sumero-Babylonia. Later excavations revealed evidence of a society in existence at least a millennium before that of the Elamites. This proto-Elamite culture, which was roughly contemporary with that of the proto-Sumerians, used numbers and linear measures virtually identical to theirs, despite a completely different style of writing.

32   Using the information in the passage, how many shu-si are in 6 nindans?

    A   180

    B   360

    C   1440

    D   2160

33 Which of the following may be safely concluded, based on information in the passage?

    1   Sexagesimal mathematical systems may have been used by more than one ancient society.

    2   Societies may use highly similar systems of numbers and measurements, yet entirely dissimilar writing styles.

A   1 only

B   2 only

C   both 1 and 2

D   neither 1 nor 2

34 The proto-Elamite society existed approximately:

A   2,800–2,900 years ago.

B   3,500–3,900 years ago.

C   4,800–4,900 years ago.

D   5,800–5,900 years ago.

35 Which one of the following, if true, would most likely challenge the interpretation about the Sumero-Babylonian number system made in the first paragraph, and explained further in the second paragraph?

A   Discovery of a Sumero-Babylonian mathematical text, revealing that the society's counting and measurement systems are based on numbers that are multiples of 6, rather than factors of 60.

B   Discovery of Sumero-Babylonian religious texts, revealing that the society's belief system involved a total of 60 gods and goddesses who controlled all aspects of life, nature and the world.

C   Discovery of a proto-Sumerian mathematical text, revealing that the proto-Sumerian counting and measurement systems were based on factors of 12, rather than factors of 60.

D   Discovery of a proto-Elamite religious text from a society that was conquered by the Sumero-Babylonians, revealing that the conquered society's belief system divided existence into 12 essential life forces.

E   Discovery of a text from the proto-Elamite school curriculum, revealing that the proto-Elamites adopted the proto-Sumerian number system after being defeated by the proto-Sumerians in a long, brutal and punishing war.

BMAT SECTION 2: SCIENTIFIC KNOWLEDGE AND APPLICATIONS (30 MINUTES)

You have 30 minutes to answer 27 questions. There are no penalties for incorrect answers, so you should attempt all questions.

Fill in your answers to each question on the answer sheet provided. Shade the circles corresponding to the answer choice(s) you have selected.

Avoid making stray marks on the paper. If you make a mistake, erase your answer completely and try again.

Calculators are **not** permitted.

1   Shown below is a haemoglobin dissociation curve, which shows what percent of the blood's haemoglobin is
     filled with oxygen at any given partial pressure of oxygen in the blood.

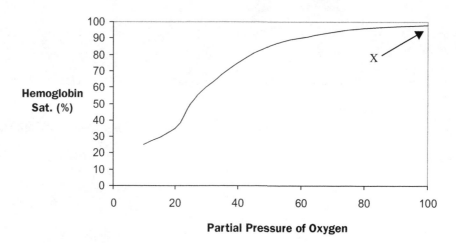

Where would you expect to find blood with characteristics matching that of point X?

A   At the end of capillaries in tissue

B   In the pulmonary vein

C   In the pulmonary artery

D   In the liver

2   A sealed system is filled with pure oxygen and 0.729 g magnesium at 25 °C, 1 atm pressure. The volume of the
     system is recorded as 10 dm^3. The magnesium is then completely combusted and the system is allowed to return
     to 25 °C, 1 atm pressure. What is the new volume of the system? Assume solids have negligible volume.

     (1 mole of any gas occupies 24 dm^3 at room temperature and pressure)

     (n.b. A_r Mg = 24.3, O = 16)

A   9.28 dm^3

B   9.64 dm^3

C   10 dm^3

D   10.36 dm^3

E   10.72 dm^3

3   What is the area of square *ABCD* if $\overline{BC}$ is its diagonal?

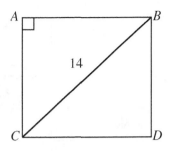

    A   28

    B   49

    C   56

    D   98

    E   196

4   A boy is travelling at 10 m/s on his bicycle when he brakes and comes to a complete stop 20 m later. The combined mass of the boy and the bicycle is 80 kg. What force is applied by the brakes?

    A   80 N

    B   160 N

    C   200 N

    D   400 N

    E   The force cannot be determined from these data alone

5   Which row of the table correctly describes what happens when a person drinks more water than necessary?

	concentration of solutes in blood	blood concentration detected by	release of ADH	concentration of solutes in urine
A	increases	hypothalamus	increases	increases
B	increases	pituitary	decreases	decreases
C	increases	cerebral cortex	increases	decreases
D	decreases	hypothalamus	decreases	decreases
E	decreases	pituitary	increases	increases
F	decreases	cerebral cortex	decreases	decreases

6   Which component is represented by X in the circuit diagram below?

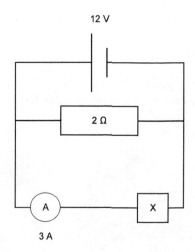

12 V

2 Ω

A

3 A

X

A   ⊢ 2 Ω ⊣

B   ⊗

C   ⊢ 4 Ω ⊣

D   ⊣⊢

E   ⊢ 6 Ω ⊣

7 In the following reaction, which statement correctly describes Au?

$$4Au\,(s) + 8\,CN-\,(aq) + O_2\,(g) + 2H_2O\,(l) \rightarrow 4\,[Au(CN_2)] - (aq) + 4OH-\,(aq)$$

A Au (s) is reduced from 0 to -1 and acts as an reducing agent.

B Au (s) is reduced from 0 to -1 and acts as an oxidising agent.

C Au (s) is oxidised from 0 to $+1$ and acts as an oxidising agent.

D Au (s) is oxidised from 0 to $+1$ and acts as an reducing agent.

E Au (s) is oxidised from 0 to $+2$ and acts as an oxidising agent.

F Au (s) is oxidised from 0 to $+2$ and acts as an reducing agent.

8 If $(36b - 35)^4 = (3b)^8$, what is one possible value of b?

A $-\dfrac{7}{3}$

B $-\dfrac{3}{5}$

C $\dfrac{1}{2}$

D $\dfrac{5}{3}$

9 Which of the following statements is true about normal running?

I The forward force of the heel strike causes a reaction force at right angles to the ground.
II The force of the toe push is balanced by a force from the ground that pushes the runner forward.
III While the runner has both feet off the ground there is no equal and opposite force to the runner's weight.

A I only

B II only

C III only

D I and II

E I and III

F II and III

10   Examine the pedigree below of a genetic disorder. If the person at the arrow has children with someone who is unaffected by the disease and is not a carrier, what are the chances that their children will be affected?

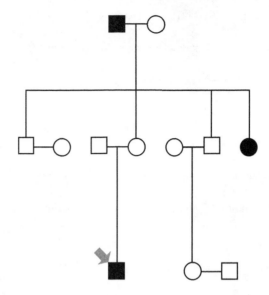

A   0%

B   25%

C   50%

D   66%

E   75%

11   In the diagram, the area of circle P is 4 times the area of circle S and $\overline{AB}$ passes through the centre of both circles. If circle S has a diameter of 8, what is the value of $\overline{AB}$?

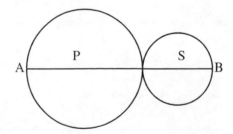

A   12

B   24

C   36

D   40

E   48

12   Copper (Cu) occurs naturally as two isotopes. ^{63}Cu has an abundance of 69%, and ^{65}Cu has an abundance of 31%.

What is the A_r of copper?

A   63.51

B   63.62

C   63.69

D   64.38

13   Which of the following features does not optimise the function of respiratory alveoli?

A   Large combined surface area

B   Delivery of environmental air to the small bronchioles by the respiratory system

C   Single layer of cells in the alveolar wall

D   Fluid coating of the alveolar wall

E   Large blood vessels coating the alveoli

14   Calcium carbonate is added in a single portion to stirred excess aqueous hydrochloric acid. The experiment is carried out under two different sets of reaction conditions, **X** and **Y**. The graph below plots the rate of CO_2 production against reaction time.

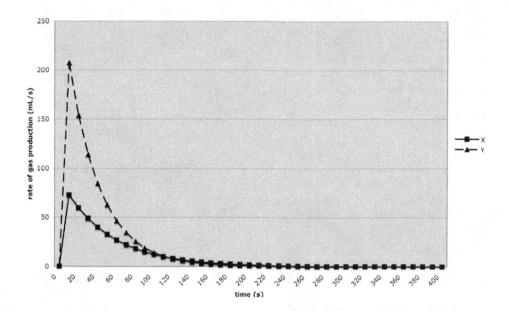

Which of the following describes changes in the reaction conditions from set **X** to set **Y**?

I   increase in the mass of $CaCO_3$

II   increase in the volume of HCl solution

III   increase in the reaction temperature

A   I only

B   II only

C   III only

D   I and II

E   I and III

F   II and III

G   I, II and III

15 A student is experimenting with her guitar, a microphone and a cathode ray oscilloscope. The oscilloscope displays the alternating current generated by the microphone when the guitar makes a sound. The student plays a note from a guitar string, and records the oscilloscope trace.

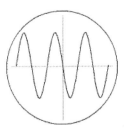

Which answer choice describes the new trace produced when the student winds the same guitar string tighter and plays a new note at the same volume?

	wavelength	amplitude	frequency
A	increases	no change	decreases
B	no change	increases	increases
C	no change	decreases	no change
D	decreases	no change	increases
E	decreases	increases	increases
F	increases	no change	increases

16 The expression $\dfrac{8x^6 - 5x^3 + 3x^2 - 7x + 9}{5x^2 + 26x - 24}$ is undefined when x is:

A $\dfrac{2}{7}$

B $\dfrac{4}{9}$

C $\dfrac{2}{3}$

D $\dfrac{4}{5}$

E $\dfrac{5}{6}$

17   Which diagram below shows a ray of light travelling from air to glass?

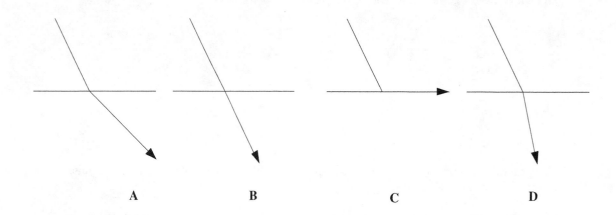

18   The following lists components of the neural and musculo-skeletal systems. Identify the correct pathway that would help a person remove their hand from a burning stove.

1. Sensory afferent nerves in the spinal cord
2. Brain
3. Sensory neuron in skin
4. Hypothalamus
5. Neuromuscular junction
6. Efferent spinal cord motor neurons

A   3 → 2 → 1 → 6 → 5

B   3 → 1 → 4 → 2 → 6

C   3 → 6 → 2 → 1 → 5

D   3 → 1 → 2 → 6 → 5

E   1 → 2 → 6 → 5 → 3

F   1 → 3 → 2 → 4 → 6

19   A reaction takes place following the steps below:

1. $CH_3CO_2H + H_2SO_4 \rightleftharpoons CH_3CO_2H_2^+ + HSO_4^-$

2. $CH_3CO_2H_2^+ + CH_3CH_2OH \rightarrow CH_3CH_2OCO_2CH_3 + H_2O + H^+$

Which of the following statements correctly describes this reaction?

1   The reaction rate is increased by the participation of H^+

2   The yield of the reaction could be improved by using ethanol as a solvent

3   The yield of the reaction could be improved by adding a substance that adsorbs water

4   The reaction product is a polymer

5   The product has no functional groups

A   1, 2 and 3

B   1, 2 and 4

C   1, 2 and 5

D   1, 3 and 4

E   1, 3 and 5

F   2, 3 and 4

G   2, 3 and 5

20   John has j 5 p coins, Katie has k 10 p coins, and Laura has l 50 p coins. The total value of the coins is £3.30. Laura realises that she would have the same amount if she combined her coins with either John or Katie. Laura sees that she has one more coin than Katie.

How many coins does Laura have?

A   3

B   4

C   5

D   6

E   7

21   In the stomach:

   I   A chemical barrier helps defend the body against microorganisms
   II   Muscular contractions help break down proteins into amino acids
   III   Fats are dispersed into tiny droplets

   A   I only

   B   II only

   C   III only

   D   I and II

   E   II and III

22   Consider the following reactions involving sodium and its compounds.

   1    $2Na + 2H_2O \rightarrow 2NaOH + H_2$
   2    $Na \rightarrow Na^+ + e^-$
   3    $4Na + O_2 \rightarrow 2Na_2O$
   4    $NaCl + AgNO_3 \rightarrow AgCl + NaNO_3$

   Which of the reactions are redox reactions?

   A   1 and 2

   B   1 and 3

   C   1 and 4

   D   2 and 3

   E   2 and 4

   F   3 and 4

23 A motor has 25% efficiency. If the motor consumes 10 W of power, how long will it take the motor to pull a 10 N brick up the wedge? ($g = 10$ m/s^2)

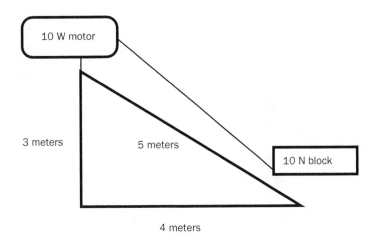

A   3 seconds

B   8 seconds

C   12 seconds

D   20 seconds

E   1 minute

24 Which of the following are correct statements about hormones?

    1   Insulin is a hormone released from the pancreas under low blood glucose levels.

    2   A hormone from the brain acts to control the water content of the blood.

    3   Some illegal drugs can increase hormone production.

    4   A hormone can affect more than one organ at once.

A   None

B   2 and 3

C   3 and 4

D   1, 2 and 3

E   1, 2 and 4

F   2, 3 and 4

G   All

25 If $5y^2 - 4x = \sqrt{4x^2 - 4x + 1}$, what is x in terms of y?

A $\quad x = \dfrac{y^2 - 1}{2}$

B $\quad x = \dfrac{5y^2 + 1}{6}$

C $\quad x = \dfrac{6}{5y^2 - 1}$

D $\quad x = \dfrac{2}{y^2}$

26 Which of the following simplified reactions occurs along the segment, in the forward direction, indicated by the arrow?

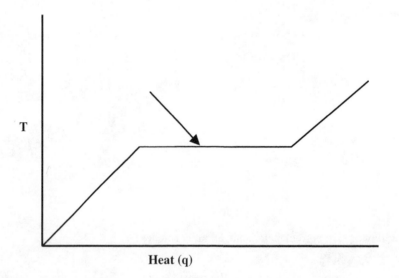

A Solid → Solid

B Solid → Liquid

C Liquid → Liquid

D Gas → Gas

E Gas → Vapour

27   A boy travels along a straight road at a velocity of 1 m/s for 10 s. He then stops for 5 s and then returns to his
       starting point at a rate of 2 m/s. Which of the following graphs represents the path of the boy?

A

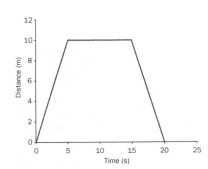

B

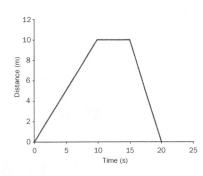

C

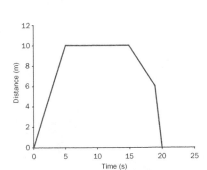

D

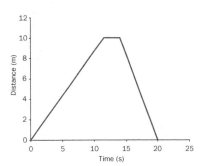

BMAT SECTION 3: WRITING TASK (30 MINUTES)

Section 3 contains a choice of three tasks. You have 30 minutes in which to answer **one**. You can take notes and make an outline in the space provided in the test booklet, but your answer must be written within the space provided on the answer sheet.

There is no correct answer to any of the questions posed. The writing task provides you with an opportunity to demonstrate your ability to:

- organise and develop your thoughts, and
- produce clear and concise written communication

Be sure to take time to organise your ideas and develop an outline. You may not use a dictionary but you may include a drawing or diagram.

Remember that you have only 30 minutes to select your task, organise your thoughts, and complete your essay.

USE THIS SPACE FOR NOTES

Answer <u>one</u> of the following questions.

1   **You must not refuse to treat a patient because their medical condition may put you at risk. If a patient poses a risk to your health or safety, you should take all available steps to minimise the risk before providing treatment or making suitable alternative arrangements for treatment.**
     (UK General Medical Council, *Good Medical Practice 2011*)

     Why are doctors required to treat patients, regardless of their medical condition? In what circumstances might a patient's medical condition make it difficult to minimise the risk to a doctor's own health and safety? How can a doctor best balance personal health and safety with that of the patient?

2   **Research is what I'm doing when I don't know what I'm doing.**
     (Wernher von Braun)

     How can the kind of research described in the quote be helpful to science? What is the advantage in research that is more directed or purposeful, and what are its limitations?

3   **Never go to a doctor whose office plants have died.**
     (Erma Bombeck)

     Can a patient expect good, reliable treatment from a doctor whose office plants have died? Explain the impact of the medical environment (doctor's office, hospital or treatment room) on patient perceptions of quality of care. What are some of the considerations doctors must make in 'keeping up appearances', so as not to undermine patient confidence?

BMAT TEST 4 – ANSWER KEY

SECTION 1	
Question	Answer
1	E
2	A
3	D
4	D
5	C
6	A
7	D
8	B
9	C
10	B
11	D
12	B
13	C
14	F
15	D
16	F
17	A
18	E
19	A
20	D
21	C
22	B
23	A
24	D
25	A
26	B
27	C
28	B
29	E
30	C
31	B
32	D
33	C
34	C
35	A

SECTION 2	
Question	Answer
1	B
2	B
3	D
4	C
5	D
6	C
7	D
8	D
9	B
10	C
11	B
12	B
13	E
14	E
15	D
16	D
17	D
18	D
19	A
20	C
21	A
22	B
23	C
24	F
25	B
26	B
27	B

BMAT TEST 4 – SCORING TABLES

1. Count up your number of correct answers in each section. Each question is worth one mark.

2. Write the total number of marks correct in each section on the lines below.

3. Find your approximate score for each section in the table below.

	NUMBER CORRECT	APPROXIMATE BMAT SCORE
Section 1	_____	_____
Section 2	_____	_____

SECTION 1		SECTION 2	
Number Correct	BMAT Score	Number Correct	BMAT Score
0	1.0	0	1.0
1	1.0	1	1.0
2	1.0	2	1.0
3	1.0	3	1.3
4	1.0	4	1.8
5	1.1	5	2.2
6	1.5	6	2.6
7	1.9	7	2.9
8	2.2	8	3.2
9	2.5	9	3.5
10	2.8	10	3.7
11	3.1	11	4.0
12	3.4	12	4.2
13	3.6	13	4.5
14	3.9	14	4.7
15	4.1	15	4.9
16	4.4	16	5.2
17	4.6	17	5.4
18	4.9	18	5.6
19	5.1	19	5.9
20	5.4	20	6.2
21	5.6	21	6.5
22	5.9	22	6.8
23	6.1	23	7.2
24	6.4	24	7.7
25	6.7	25	8.3
26	7.0	26	9.0
27	7.3	27	9.0
28	7.6		
29	8.0		
30	8.4		
31	8.9		
32	9.0		
33	9.0		
34	9.0		
35	9.0		

N.B. These scores are for approximation purposes only. The scoring tables used for the BMAT vary slightly year to year, depending on student performance and the norming of the questions in each version of the test paper. To err on the side of caution, these scoring tables are among the toughest ever used on the BMAT. In most cases, a similar performance on the BMAT would result in a slightly higher score.

Test 5

BMAT
Section 1

Test ID

Test 1 ○ Test 2 ○ Test 3 ○ Test 4 ○ Test 5 ●

Last Name

First Name

Date

Completely fill in the space for your intended answer choice

A B C D E
○ ○ ● ○ ○

1   A B C D E F G H
    ○ ○ ○ ○ ○ ○ ○ ○

2   A B C D E
    ○ ○ ○ ○ ○

3   A B C D
    ○ ○ ○ ○

4   A B C D
    ○ ○ ○ ○

5   A B C D
    ○ ○ ○ ○

6   A B C D E F
    ○ ○ ○ ○ ○ ○

7   A B C D E
    ○ ○ ○ ○ ○

8   A B C D E
    ○ ○ ○ ○ ○

9   A B C D E
    ○ ○ ○ ○ ○

10 A B C D
    ○ ○ ○ ○

11 A B C D
    ○ ○ ○ ○

12 A B C D E
    ○ ○ ○ ○ ○

13 A B C D
    ○ ○ ○ ○

14 A B C D E
    ○ ○ ○ ○ ○

15 A B C D E
    ○ ○ ○ ○ ○

16 A B C D E
    ○ ○ ○ ○ ○

17 A B C D E
    ○ ○ ○ ○ ○

18 A B C D
    ○ ○ ○ ○

19 A B C D E
    ○ ○ ○ ○ ○

20 A B C D
    ○ ○ ○ ○

21 A B C D
    ○ ○ ○ ○

22 A B C D E
    ○ ○ ○ ○ ○

23 A B C D E
    ○ ○ ○ ○ ○

24 A B C D E
    ○ ○ ○ ○ ○

25 A B C D E F
    ○ ○ ○ ○ ○ ○

26 A B C D E
    ○ ○ ○ ○ ○

27 A B C D E
    ○ ○ ○ ○ ○

28 A B C D
    ○ ○ ○ ○

29 A B C D E
    ○ ○ ○ ○ ○

30 A B C D E
    ○ ○ ○ ○ ○

31 A B C D E
    ○ ○ ○ ○ ○

32 A B C D E
    ○ ○ ○ ○ ○

33 A B C D E
    ○ ○ ○ ○ ○

34 A B C D E
    ○ ○ ○ ○ ○

35 A B C D E
    ○ ○ ○ ○ ○

BMAT is a registered trademark of Cambridge Assessment, which neither sponsors nor endorses this product.

K 193

BMAT
Section 2

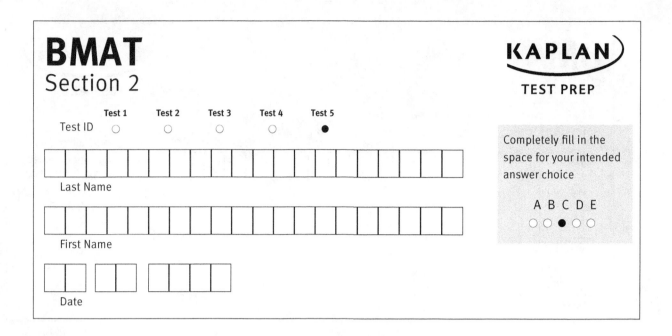

Test ID

Test 1 ○ Test 2 ○ Test 3 ○ Test 4 ○ Test 5 ●

Last Name

First Name

Date

Completely fill in the space for your intended answer choice

A B C D E
○ ○ ● ○ ○

1 A B C D E
   ○ ○ ○ ○ ○

2 A B C D
   ○ ○ ○ ○

3 A B C D E
   ○ ○ ○ ○ ○

4 A B C D
   ○ ○ ○ ○

5 A B C D E F G H
   ○ ○ ○ ○ ○ ○ ○ ○

6 A B C D
   ○ ○ ○ ○

7 A B C D
   ○ ○ ○ ○

8 A B C D E
   ○ ○ ○ ○ ○

9 A B C D
   ○ ○ ○ ○

10 A B C D
    ○ ○ ○ ○

11 A B C D E
    ○ ○ ○ ○ ○

12 A B C D E
    ○ ○ ○ ○ ○

13 A B C D E
    ○ ○ ○ ○ ○

14 A B C D
    ○ ○ ○ ○

15 A B C D E
    ○ ○ ○ ○ ○

16 A B C D E F
    ○ ○ ○ ○ ○ ○

17 A B C D
    ○ ○ ○ ○

18 A B C D E
    ○ ○ ○ ○ ○

19 A B C D
    ○ ○ ○ ○

20 A B C D E F
    ○ ○ ○ ○ ○ ○

21 A B C D
    ○ ○ ○ ○

22 A B C D E
    ○ ○ ○ ○ ○

23 A B C D E
    ○ ○ ○ ○ ○

24 A B C D E F G
    ○ ○ ○ ○ ○ ○ ○

25 A B C D
    ○ ○ ○ ○

26 A B C D E F
    ○ ○ ○ ○ ○ ○

27 A B C D E
    ○ ○ ○ ○ ○

BMAT
Section 3

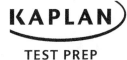

	Test 1	Test 2	Test 3	Test 4	Test 5	Test 6
Test ID	○	○	○	○	○	○

Last Name

First Name

Question answered ☐

Your answer must be contained within this area.

BMAT is a registered trademark of Cambridge Assessment, which neither sponsors nor endorses this product.

195

BMAT SECTION 1: APTITUDE AND SKILLS (60 MINUTES)

You have 60 minutes to answer 35 questions. There are no penalties for incorrect answers, so you should attempt all questions.

Fill in your answers to each question on the answer sheet provided. Shade the circles corresponding to the answer choice(s) you have selected.

Avoid making stray marks on the paper. If you make a mistake, erase your answer completely and try again.

Calculators are **not** permitted.

1   Data about crime rates for Lincoln, and for the entire UK, in 2005–2006 is given in the table below.

Offence	Total Locally	Per 1000 Population	
		Locally	Nationally
Robbery	73	0.84	1.85
Theft of a motor vehicle	283	3.27	4.04
Theft from a motor vehicle	789	9.12	9.56
Sexual offences	186	2.15	1.17
Violence against a person	2885	33.33	19.97
Burglary	552	6.38	5.67
TOTAL	4768		
		Local	National
	POPULATION	86,547	60,200,000
	HOUSEHOLDS	37,000	24,900,000

Which of the following statements about crimes in 2005–2006 can be correctly inferred from the data above?

1   There were more burglaries locally than nationally.
2   Approximately 60% of local crimes involved violence against a person.
3   The national rate of robberies was more than twice the local rate.
4   Most crimes committed nationally involved violence against a person.

A   1 and 2

B   1 and 3

C   1 and 4

D   2 and 3

E   2 and 4

F   3 and 4

G   1, 2 and 3

H   1, 3 and 4

2   Ordering books online is the best option for all customers who love saving money as much as they love reading. Book retailers that operate online are able to offer an extensive range of titles, including all the popular books of the day and many other titles that can be difficult for bookshops to stock, and it is a major inconvenience for customers to have to wait while a bookshop locates, orders and secures delivery of such books. This is the sort of time-consuming procedure one might expect for obscure or specialist titles, not for the books that everyone is reading! Online book retailers are also able to offer significant discounts from the recommended retail price for most titles, as these retailers operate with significantly reduced overhead as compared to traditional high street bookshops.

Which one of the following, if true, would be most likely to weaken the argument above?

A   Online book retailers sell a greater range of titles than any high street bookshop.

B   Some online book retailers are owned and operated by companies known for their high street bookshops.

C   Books that everyone is reading can be bought easily at any high street bookshop.

D   Books that everyone is reading are discounted an average of 25% at online book retailers.

E   Many cost-conscious readers want to buy obscure or specialist titles that are not listed by online book retailers.

3   A set of double-nine dominoes includes a total of 55 dominoes. Each domino is divided into two segments, and each segment has a total of 0 to 9 dots. Every possible pair of numbers from 0 to 9 occurs exactly once in the set. What is the total number of dots on all the dominoes in the set?

A   480

B   495

C   510

D   525

4   Aisling is preparing to make soup. She has 4 carrots for every 3 swedes, 12 beans for every 2 swedes, and 1 tomato for every 15 beans. What is the ratio of carrots to tomatoes?

A   10 : 3

B   5 : 2

C   4 : 1

D   3 : 5

Questions 5 and 6 refer to the information in the table and paragraph below.

PEDESTRIAN CASUALTIES IN THE UK, 2001–2009

Killed by cycles	18
Seriously injured by cycles	434
Killed by cars	3,495
Seriously injured by cars	46,245

In 2008, a total of 13,272 collisions between cars and cycles were recorded in the UK. These collisions resulted in the deaths of a total of 52 cyclists, but no deaths of people inside the cars (drivers or passengers) that were involved. A study of all collisions involving cycles and cars from the prior three years revealed that police determined that car drivers were to blame in 60% of such collisions, that cyclists were to blame in 30% of such collisions and that both car driver and cyclist were jointly to blame in 10% of such collisions.

5   What percentage of pedestrians killed or seriously injured by cars or cycles in the UK from 2001–2009 were killed by cars?

   A   3.5%

   B   5%

   C   7%

   D   9.5%

6   Which of the following can be most properly inferred from the information?

   1   Passengers in cars are unlikely to die in collisions with cycles.
   2   Drivers of cars cause more collisions than cyclists.
   3   Pedestrians should not worry about being killed by cyclists.

   A   1 only

   B   2 only

   C   1 and 2

   D   1 and 3

   E   2 and 3

   F   1, 2 and 3

7   Marisia: Maths should not be compulsory for GCSEs, because skills involving maths are not of practical use in most people's daily lives, beyond basic calculations which can be done with a calculator.

Shabnam: But you are ignoring the fact that some of the most practical accomplishments in human history would have been impossible without more advanced maths. For example, without trigonometry, we would not be able to sail across large bodies of water, or build structurally sound houses.

Which one of the following most clearly states the conclusion of Shabnam's argument?

A   Trigonometry should be compulsory for GCSEs.

B   Maths does have some practical uses.

C   People who work in sailing and construction need to know trigonometry.

D   Only skills required in daily life should be compulsory for GCSEs.

E   Everyone uses maths in daily life.

8   If folded up, the pattern below will form a cube.

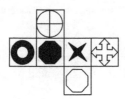

Which one of the following patterns could fold up to form an identical cube?

A

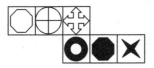

B

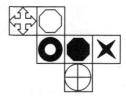

C

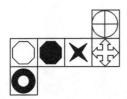

D

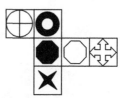

E

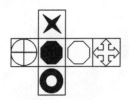

Questions 9 to 12 refer to the following information.

A survey of UK workers in 2009 asked how long they spent traveling to work in their daily commute, and how they commuted to work. Results are given in the graphs below.

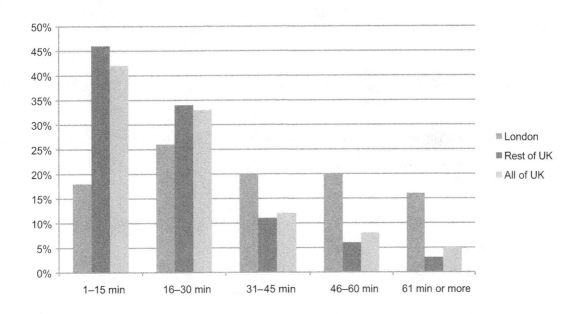

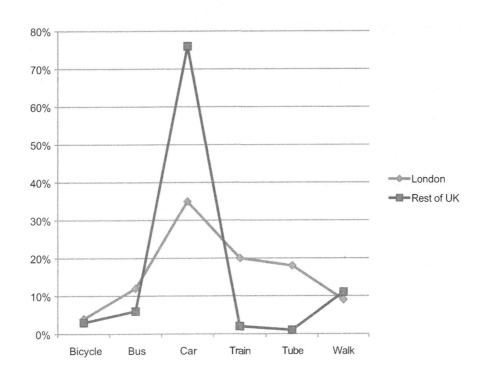

In 2009, the UK had a total population of 61,194,500. The population of London was 12.7% of the UK total in 2009.

The survey also compared certain information about workers with long commutes (61 minutes or more) and workers with short commutes (1 to 15 minutes). Workers with long commutes earned an average of £18.80 per hour in London (and £14.30 in the rest of the UK), while workers with short commutes earned an average of £9.60 per hour in London (and £8.30 in the rest of the UK). The survey also found that 29% of people in full-time work and 14% of people in part-time work had long commutes, and that 36% of people in managerial and professional jobs and 12% of people in low-skill work had long commutes. Thus, one can conclude that higher salaries and higher-skilled jobs are connected with long commutes, rather than with short commutes.

9   Which one of the following can be safely concluded about commutes to work in the UK in 2009, based on the data?

   A   Ten times as many workers traveled to work by train in London as in the rest of the UK.

   B   Four times as many workers had commutes of over an hour in London as in the rest of the UK.

   C   60% of workers in the UK traveled to work by car.

   D   80% of workers in the UK had commutes of 30 minutes or less.

   E   More workers walked to work in the rest of the UK than in London.

10   What was the population of London in 2009?

   A   6,892,400

   B   7,185,200

   C   7,774,600

   D   8,363,100

11   How many workers in the UK had commutes of 30 minutes or less in 2009?

   A   44,671,985

   B   45,895,875

   C   46,705,280

   D   48,955,600

12   Which one of the following, if true, would be most likely to support the claim about the salaries of workers with long commutes?

    A   Workers with short commutes have more children, on average, than workers with long commutes.

    B   Workers with long commutes are more likely to live in London than in the rest of the UK.

    C   Workers with long commutes are more likely to travel to work by car than workers with short commutes.

    D   Workers with long commutes have a higher standard and cost of living than workers with short commutes.

    E   Workers with short commutes earn less per hour than workers with long commutes.

13   After going on the market in January, the price of a house increases by 8% in February, and by another 5% in March. The price of the house is £567,000 at the end of March. What was its original price in January?

    A   £480,000

    B   £495,500

    C   £500,000

    D   £512,250

14   Dr Brennan is one of the most respected neuro-oncologists in the country, and a long waiting list of people with brain tumours want him to become their doctor. These people should think twice, however, because a high percentage of Dr Brennan's patients die during or just after surgery. A much higher percentage of Dr Sonjay's patients survive and recover.

Which **one** of the following, if true, most weakens the above argument?

    A   Dr Sonjay thinks that Dr Brennan deserves to be respected as a neuro-oncologist.

    B   Many patients who are on a waiting list for Dr Brennan have met with Dr Sonjay.

    C   Dr Brennan regularly performs operations that entail a high level of risk.

    D   Dr Brennan has been a practicing neuro-oncologist for much longer than Dr Sonjay has.

    E   Dr Brennan has a better track record than many neuro-oncologists, though not better than Dr Sonjay.

15   The graph shows the number of cars sold by company *A* and company *B* in the years 2001, 2002, 2003 and 2004. Which of the three statements can be deduced from the information?

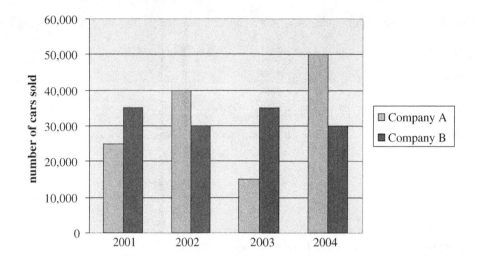

1   The number of cars sold by company A in any of the years shown was never more than twice the number of cars sold by company B.

2   The total number of cars sold by company A in the years 2003 and 2004 was less than the total number of cars sold by company B in the years 2003 and 2004.

3   The percent increase in the number of cars sold by company A from 2003 to 2004 was less than 300%.

A   1 only

B   3 only

C   1 and 2 only

D   1 and 3 only

E   All

16   Alborne is north of Millerton and south of Creighton. Dourbon is north of Feltshire, which is south of Creighton.

Therefore, Alborne must be south of:

A   Dourbon, but not necessarily Creighton or Feltshire;

B   Feltshire, but not necessarily Dourbon or Millerton;

C   Millerton, but not Creighton and not necessarily Dourbon;

D   Creighton, but not necessarily Dourbon or Feltshire;

E   Feltshire, Dourbon and Creighton.

17   Over the past six months there has been an increase in seismic activity in the vicinity of a certain volcano. Therefore, the evacuation plan for the burgeoning communities nearby is inadequate to protect the population and a new plan should be put into place as soon as possible.

Which of the following are underlying assumptions of the above argument?

1   An increase in seismic activity in the vicinity of the volcano indicates that the volcano may erupt.

2   The current evacuation plan is inadequate to protect the population of the neighbouring communities.

3   The population of the neighbouring communities can be protected from a volcanic eruption with an adequate evacuation plan.

A   1 only

B   1 and 2 only

C   1 and 3 only

D   2 and 3 only

E   1, 2 and 3

18   A comet first appears in 1917, and then re-appears every four years. In what year will the comet make its 53rd appearance?

A   2117

B   2125

C   2129

D   2137

19   Whale-watching has become a lucrative sector within the tourist industry, which is taken up by some 13 million people each year and is worth over a £1 billion. However, the increase in whale-watching has been extremely harmful to whales, whose feeding and parenting habits are disrupted by the continued presence of boats in their waters. As a result, pods of whales have been documented as raising far fewer offspring successfully to full maturity in many areas where whale-watching tours are heavily subscribed, than in areas where whale-watching is banned. Thus, it's obvious that whale-watching is the greatest harm to whales today, and should be banned worldwide.

Which one of the following, if true, would represent the best attack against the argument above?

A   Whales that grow accustomed to being watched by tourists are not interested in parenting their offspring.

B   All the major whale-watching tour companies invest a share of their profits in preserving whale habitats.

C   People are more likely to donate to environmental causes after going on a whale-watching tour.

D   Pollution of the oceans prevents more whales worldwide from surviving to maturity than any other cause.

E   Whales develop elaborate daily routines with their offspring in areas where whale-watching is banned.

Questions 20 to 23 refer to the information below.

The graph below indicates the population of the local authorities in the UK that experienced the greatest percentage rise in population from 1999 to 2009.

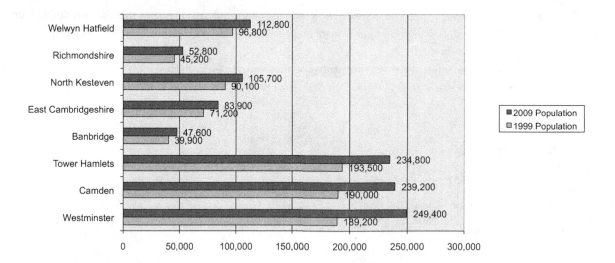

The three local authority areas that experienced the greatest percentage rise and the greatest absolute rise in population from 1999 to 2009 – Westminster, Camden and Tower Hamlets – are all located in central London. Two of the other local authorities – Welwyn Hatfield in Hertfordshire, and East Cambridgeshire in Cambridgeshire – are within an hour of London. The remaining local authorities are in the East Midlands (North Kesteven), Yorkshire (Richmondshire) or Northern Ireland (Banbridge). Almost all of the remaining local authorities in the UK that experienced positive population growth from 1999 to 2009 are in England.

20   The population of Westminster rose by what percentage?

A   24%

B   26%

C   30%

D   32%

21   Which of the following statements can be safely inferred from the information above?

    1   The only UK local authority to grow by more than 50,000 people from 1999 to 2009 was in London.

    2   England experienced positive population growth from 1999 to 2009.

    A   1 only

    B   2 only

    C   both 1 and 2

    D   neither 1 nor 2

22   Which local authority outside London experienced the greatest percentage growth in population?

    A   Welwyn Hatfield

    B   Richmondshire

    C   North Kesteven

    D   East Cambridgeshire

    E   Banbridge

23   Politician: These population statistics show a shocking growth in the number of people living in central London, where demand on housing has driven the cost of living to unreasonable proportions. The rise in central London's population is not due to people having more children, as birth rates are declining in London and across the UK. The only solution to deal with this population explosion and make London livable and affordable is to impose strict limits on immigration to the UK.

Which one of the following, if true, would be most likely to weaken the politician's argument?

    A   The vast majority of people who moved to central London from 1999 to 2009 relocated from outside the UK.

    B   The vast majority of people who moved to central London from 1999 to 2009 relocated from other parts of the UK.

    C   People living in central London from 1999 to 2009 had significantly more children in those years than people in other parts of the UK.

    D   Many people moved from outer London to central London between 1999 and 2009.

    E   Many people moved from central London to outer London between 1999 and 2009.

24   Liam is making pancakes for a big brunch. He needs to make a total of 80 pancakes, and can make 4 at a time on his hob. It takes Liam 3 minutes to mix a batch of batter, which will make a total of 15 pancakes. Cooking the pancakes takes 7 minutes, and Liam can mix a new batch of batter if needed while pancakes are cooking on the hob. Once pancakes are finished cooking, Liam must let the pans cool for 5 minutes before starting to cook more pancakes. If Liam starts at 7am, at what time will he finish?

    A   10.55am

    B   10.58am

    C   11.00am

    D   11.03am

    E   11.08am

25   A lottery involves selecting a 4-digit number, from 0000 to 9999, using 4 sets of balls numbered from 0 to 9. The 4 numbers are selected independently and randomly. What is the probability that all 4 digits in the number selected will be different?

    A $\dfrac{42}{125}$

    B $\dfrac{56}{125}$

    C $\dfrac{12}{25}$

    D $\dfrac{63}{125}$

    E $\dfrac{14}{25}$

    F $\dfrac{7}{10}$

26   A magazine has a policy that prohibits its employees from personal use of company computers. But the IT department is too small to adequately enforce this policy, and most employees check their personal email at work each day. If the policy were rescinded, the IT department could spend more time on efficiency-improving projects such as training and maintenance. Clearly, the magazine should rescind the policy.

Which **one** of the following, if true, most undermines the argument above?

A   Most employees currently check their personal email quickly and efficiently.

B   The policy reduces personal use of company computers.

C   None of the employees has expressed interest in training done by the IT department.

D   The employees who most resent the policy are those who are most likely to break it.

E   The policy does not prevent personal use of company computers.

27   A code is expressed as a line of 5 colours in a particular order. The colours can be chosen from the following list: red, blue, green, grey, black, yellow and orange. A colour may only be used once in a code. Colours with the same initial letter are not permitted in the same code.

The first attempt to reproduce 'Code X' was as follows:

1 black 2 orange 3 red 4 yellow 5 grey

It is known that 2 and 5 are correct, but that 1, 3 and 4 are incorrect.

Which **one** of the following attempts at Code X **may** be correct?

A   1 red 2 orange 3 green 4 yellow 5 grey

B   1 yellow 2 orange 3 red 4 blue 5 grey

C   1 blue   2 orange 3 yellow 4 black 5 grey

D   1 red 2 orange 3 yellow 4 blue 5 grey

E   1 black 2 orange 3 yellow 4 red 5 grey

28 The graphs below illustrate how the speeds of ascent of four different hot-air balloons (H, I, J and K) vary over a period of 120 seconds.

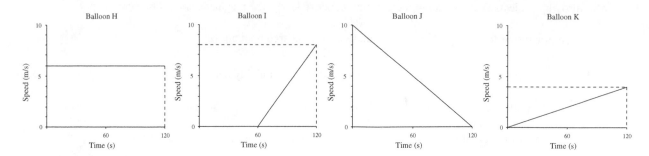

Which of the two balloons gained the same altitude in 120 seconds?

A   H and I

B   H and J

C   I and K

D   J and K

29 Recent studies suggest that mobile phone users talk more while driving than while doing any other activity. This is an increasingly serious threat to public safety. Drivers are distracted by their conversations, but they are even more distracted by all the attendant peripheral activities, such as finding the phone when it rings, or dialling. We should therefore support legislation that restricts mobile phone use on the road.

Which **one** of the following, if true, most strengthens the above argument?

A   Mobile phone use by passengers will not pose a threat to public safety.

B   Laws that reduce a threat to public safety should be supported.

C   Some level of distraction while driving is acceptable.

D   The only way to avoid serious threats to public safety is to pass laws.

E   Mobile phone users will be reluctant to stop using their phones while driving.

30 A game is played by spinning the arrow on the circular game board below. The spinner is an arrow of length 2 attached to the centre of the circle. The perpendicular distance between the centre of the circle and the line dividing the win and lose zones is $\sqrt{3}$.

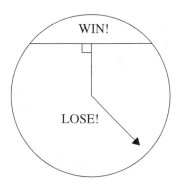

The spinner is hit sufficiently hard so that the direction it points after it has stopped spinning is random and every orientation is equally probable. What is the probability that the spinner lands in the win zone?

A 1/6

B 1/3

C 1/2

D $1/\sqrt{3}$

E 5/6

31 Becoming a successful professional athlete requires natural talent and the ability to train rigorously. My sister, an extremely talented runner, has demonstrated that she can train rigorously. So I'm certain that she can succeed as a professional athlete.

The argument above is most vulnerable to which **one** of the following criticisms?

A It depends on an imprecise use of the term 'talent'.

B It fails to consider how rigorously one must train in order to succeed as a professional runner.

C It confuses what is necessary for a situation to occur with what is sufficient to guarantee that situation.

D It assumes that the sister wants to become a professional athlete.

E It assumes that no professional athlete can succeed without natural talent.

Question 32 to 35 refer to the following information:

The table below shows the total sales and the number of items sold by two groups of employees who work for the same company.

| | Group 1 | | | Group 2 | |
Employee	Total sales for the previous month (£)	Number of items sold	Employee	Total sales for the previous month (£)	Number of items sold
Salesperson A	12,000	18	Salesperson H	14,000	21
Salesperson B	14,000	20	Salesperson I	26,000	50
Salesperson C	31,000	35	Salesperson J	42,000	31
Salesperson D	24,000	36	Salesperson K	21,000	26
Salesperson E	23,000	14	Salesperson L	15,000	24
Salesperson F	28,000	23	Salesperson M	46,000	31
Salesperson G	41,000	24	Salesperson N	31,000	14
Total	172,000	170	**Total**	195,000	197

32   What was the average of the number of items sold in the previous month by sales person N and all the members of Group 1?

A   23

B   26

C   28

D   30

E   31

33   What was the average sales amount per item, in pounds, for all the items sold by both groups?

A   500

B   750

C   1,000

D   1,125

E   1,835.50

34   If the total sales for group 1 this month are 20% greater than in the previous month, and the total sales for group 2 are 10% greater than in the previous month, what will the total sales of both groups be in this month, in pounds?

    A   403,700

    B   410,900

    C   412,875

    D   422,050

    E   430,400

35   Based on results from the previous month, the salesperson with the greatest total sales in each group is switched to the other group, and the total number of items sold are then recalculated for the new groups. Which of the new groups will have sold more items in the previous month, and how many more items will they have sold?

    A   Group 1; 1 more item

    B   Group 1; 7 more items

    C   Group 2; 7 more items

    D   Group 2; 13 more items

    E   Group 2; 47 more items

BMAT SECTION 2: SCIENTIFIC KNOWLEDGE AND APPLICATIONS (30 MINUTES)

You have 30 minutes to answer 27 questions. There are no penalties for incorrect answers, so you should attempt all questions.

Fill in your answers to each question on the answer sheet provided. Shade the circles corresponding to the answer choice(s) you have selected.

Avoid making stray marks on the paper. If you make a mistake, erase your answer completely and try again.

Calculators are **not** permitted.

1   Organs of the digestive system include:

  (i)   salivary glands

  (ii) oesophagus

  (iii) stomach

  (iv) liver

  (v)   pancreas

  (vi) small intestine

  (vii) large intestine

Which of these organs assist in the enzymatic breakdown of food?

A   (i)   (iii)   (v)   (vi)

B   (ii)   (iii)   (iv)   (vi)

C   (i)   (ii)   (v)   (vii)

D   (iii)   (iv)   (v)   (vi)

E   (iii)   (v)   (vi)   (vii)

2   What is the area of $\varnothing FGH$?

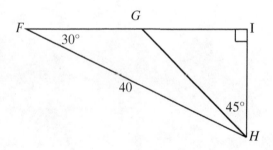

A   200

B $200\sqrt{3} - 200$

C $200\sqrt{3}$

D $200\sqrt{3} + 200$

3   The multistage rocket shown below is at rest in deep space. Each of the three components has equal mass. To propel the capsule (represented by a triangle) forward, the two tanks are launched with a speed v (as measured by an observer at rest).

Before:

After:

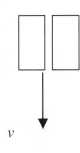

v

What is the final speed of the space capsule?

A   1/3 v

B   1/2 v

C v

D   4/3 v

E   2v

4   What mass of dissolved KOH would be needed to neutralise 500 cm^3 of 0.050 mol/dm^3 aqueous solution of a diprotic acid?

(M$_r$ of KOH = 56)

A   0.35 g

B   0.7 g

C   1.4 g

D   2.8 g

5   Regarding the Group 1 elements in the periodic table:

1   Each of these elements reacts with water to form an acidic solution and hydrogen gas.
2   Each of these elements is a metal.
3   Each of these elements reacts with oxygen to form an oxide.
4   Hydrogen is not one of these elements.

Which statements are correct?

A   1 and 2

B   2 and 3

C   3 and 4

D   1, 2 and 3

E   1, 2 and 4

F   1, 3 and 4

G   2, 3 and 4

H   All

Below are two diagrams representing the volume of the lungs and intra alveolar pressure during a single cycle of inspiration and expiration.

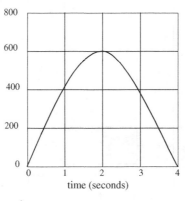

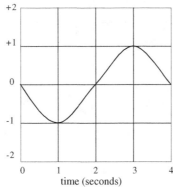

6   At which time is the velocity of exhaled air the greatest?

    A   1 seconds

    B   2 seconds

    C   3 seconds

    D   4 seconds

7   What is the equivalent resistance for the circuit?

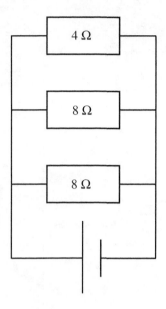

A   1 Ω

B   2 Ω

C   7 Ω

D   14 Ω

8   Which of the following is NOT a factor of $\left(9^{\frac{3}{8}} \times 7^{\frac{3}{4}} \right)^{4}$?

A   3

B   7

C   21

D   23

E   27

9   The Haber Process is a method of producing ammonia, described below. What effect will increasing the volume of the container have on the Haber Process?

$$N_2(g) + 3H_2(g) \rightarrow 2NH_3(g) \qquad \oslash H = -92.4 \text{ kJ/mole}$$

A   Reactants will be favoured.

B   Products will be favoured.

C   Neither products nor reactants will be favoured.

D   Products will be hydrolysed.

10   The amount of blood pumped by the heart per minute is called the cardiac output. It is affected by both the stroke volume, the amount of blood pumped with each heartbeat, and by the number of heartbeats per minute (heart rate). Which of the following equations most likely represents the relationship between the cardiac output (CO), stroke volume (SV) and heart rate (HR)?

A $SV/HR = CO$

B $SV = CO/HR$

C $SV + HR = CO$

D   None of the above

11   Which of the following is NOT equal to $5 + \dfrac{13}{17}$?

A $6 - \dfrac{4}{17}$

B $\dfrac{170}{34} + \dfrac{26}{35}$

C $\dfrac{49}{6} \times \dfrac{12}{17}$

D $\dfrac{6 + \dfrac{1}{8}}{1 + \dfrac{1}{16}}$

E $\dfrac{98}{17}$

12   A ball with mass m is dropped from a height of 5 metres. What is the velocity of the ball just before it hits the ground? (Assume gravity to be 10 m/s^2.)

   A   1 m/s

   B   2 m/s

   C   9 m/s

   D   10 m/s

   E   cannot be determined

13   The reaction below takes place in aqueous solution.

$$wC_6H_{12}O_6 \text{ (aq)} + xO_2 \text{ (aq)} \rightarrow yCO_2 \text{ (aq)} + zH_2O \text{ (l)}$$

What are the values of w, x, y and z?

	w	x	y	z
A	1	6	6	6
B	2	18	12	12
C	1	9	6	6
D	1	9	6	6
E	2	12	12	6

14   Which of the following correctly traces the path of oxygen as it moves into the bloodstream during inspiration?

   A   trachea → bronchi → bronchioles → alveoli → capillary

   B   capillary → trachea → bronchioles → bronchi → alveoli

   C   trachea → bronchioles → bronchi → alveoli → capillary

   D   capillary → bronchi → bronchioles → alveoli → trachea

15   A square of side z is inscribed with a vertex at the origin of a circle of radius z.

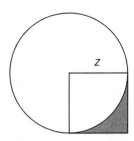

The area of the shaded area is $25(4 - \pi)$. What is the area of the circle?

A π

B   4

C 25π

D   100

E 100π

16   The diagram shows a beam of light entering a prism.

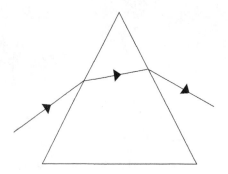

Which row of the table correctly identifies which of the speed, frequency and wavelength of the wave changes when the wave changes direction?

	speed	wavelength	frequency
A	no change	no change	no change
B	change	no change	no change
C	no change	change	change
D	change	change	change
E	no change	no change	change
F	change	change	no change

17   The reaction below describes the conversion of sodium azide to nitrogen gas.

$$2NaN_3 \ (s) \rightarrow 2Na \ (s) + 3 \ N_2 \ (g)$$

If 4.5 moles of nitrogen gas are produced, then what is the mass of sodium that is produced?

(n.b. A_r Na = 23)

A   15.3 g

B   46 g

C   69 g

D   103.5 g

18   At the instant of firing, the velocity of a cannonball can be represented by the vector v, which is inclined at θ degrees from the horizontal.

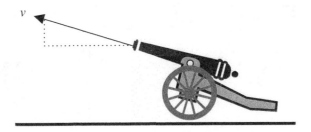

Which answer choice expresses the vertical component of the velocity?

A v

B $v \sin \theta$

C $v \cos \theta$

D $\dfrac{v^2}{2}$

E   0

19    $(x + 1) \times 10^x + (2x + 1) \times 10^{x-1} = 8300000$

What is the value of x?

A   2

B   6

C   8

D   12

20   Which row of the table correctly describes the human digestive responses to eating food?

	pH of stomach secretions	gut peristalsis	hormones to regulate appetite
A	increases	decreases	inhibitory
B	no change	no change	no change
C	increases	decreases	stimulatory
D	decreases	increases	inhibitory
E	decreases	decreases	stimulatory
F	no change	increases	no change

21   Which of the following is the formula for iron(III) sulphate?

A Fe_3SO_4

B $Fe_2(SO_4)_2$

C $Fe_2(SO_4)_3$

D $Fe3(SO_4)^3$

22   In the diagram below, the apparatus accelerates at a rate of 4 m/s2.

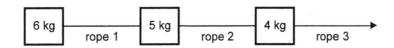

What is the tension in each of the numbered ropes?

	rope 1	rope 2	rope 3
A	40 N	50 N	60 N
B	60 N	44N	24 N
C	24 N	20 N	16 N
D	60 N	60 N	60 N
E	24 N	44 N	60 N

23   In the diagram, A is the midpoint of $\overline{WY}$. If the area of rectangle $WYZX$ is 48, what is the area of the unshaded region?

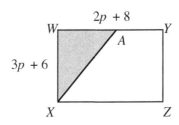

A   12

B   24

C   36

D   48

E   72

24   Below is a simplified representation of a human nephron.

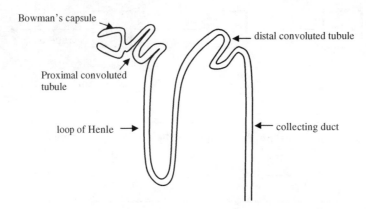

Which of the following statements correctly describes the function of the nephron?

1   Water, urea, ions and sugar are filtered into Bowman's capsule.

2   The kidney releases ADH into the collecting duct to control the concentration of urine.

3   Ions are reabsorbed in the nephron to control the level of salts in the blood.

A   1 only

B   2 only

C   3 only

D   1 and 2

E   1 and 3

F   2 and 3

G   1, 2 and 3

25   Object *A* is at a higher temperature than object *B*. When they are placed in contact, heat is transferred from object *A* to object *B*. As heat is transferred, the temperature of object *B* must:

A   Increase

B   Decrease

C   Remain the same

D   Cannot be determined

26   Consider the following circuit.

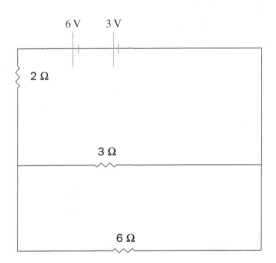

After the circuit runs for a few minutes, the 6 ohm resistor melts (it was defective), leaving that part of the circuit open. What happens to current in the 3 ohm resistor?

A   It remains the same.

B   It decreases by 1.8 A.

C   It decreases by 0.3 A.

D   It increases by 0.3 A.

E   It increases by 1.5 A.

F   It drops to zero.

27   Which one of the following correctly completes the statement?

In the synthesis of _____ to unwind and unzip.

A   amino acids, RNA causes the ribosome

B   proteins, enzymes cause DNA

C   DNA, enzymes cause proteins

D   enzymes, mitochondria cause DNA

E   proteins, ribosomes cause RNA

BMAT SECTION 3: WRITING TASK (30 MINUTES)

Section 3 contains a choice of three tasks. You have 30 minutes in which to answer **one**. You can take notes and make an outline in the space provided in the test booklet, but your answer must be written within the space provided on the answer sheet.

There is no correct answer to any of the questions posed. The writing task provides you with an opportunity to demonstrate your ability to:

- organise and develop your thoughts, and
- produce clear and concise written communication

Be sure to take time to organise your ideas and develop an outline. You may not use a dictionary but you may include a drawing or diagram.

Remember that you have only 30 minutes to select your task, organise your thoughts, and complete your essay.

Answer <u>one</u> of the following questions.

1   **All essential prescription medicines should be provided to patients free of charge.**

Is it ethical to charge patients for prescription medicines? Argue the opposite of the quotation; that is, make the case for the reasons why and how patients should be charged for essential prescription medicines.

2   **Science is a cemetery of dead ideas.**

(Miguel de Unamuno)

Explain what is meant by this quotation, using an example of a scientific 'dead idea'. Defend science as a living, growing body of knowledge, then explain how such 'dead ideas' contribute to it.

3   **We have not lost faith, but we have transferred it from God to the medical profession.**

(George Bernard Shaw)

Give an example of a circumstance in which people might be said to have 'faith' in doctors. How is this similar to (or different from) faith of a religious nature? How does it help to think of patients' views of doctors in terms of faith?

BMAT TEST 5 – ANSWER KEY

SECTION 1		SECTION 2	
Question	Answer	Question	Answer
1	D	1	A
2	E	2	B
3	B	3	E
4	A	4	C
5	C	5	G
6	A	6	C
7	B	7	B
8	E	8	D
9	E	9	A
10	C	10	B
11	B	11	B
12	D	12	D
13	C	13	A
14	C	14	A
15	D	15	E
16	D	16	F
17	C	17	C
18	B	18	B
19	D	19	B
20	D	20	D
21	A	21	C
22	E	22	E
23	B	23	C
24	B	24	E
25	D	25	D
26	B	26	D
27	D	27	B
28	C		
29	B		
30	A		
31	C		
32	A		
33	C		
34	B		
35	D		

BMAT TEST 5 – SCORING TABLES

1. Count up your number of correct answers in each section. Each question is worth one mark.
2. Write the total number of marks correct in each section on the lines below.
3. Find your approximate score for each section in the table below.

	NUMBER CORRECT	APPROXIMATE BMAT SCORE
Section 1	_____	_____
Section 2	_____	_____

SECTION 1	
Number Correct	BMAT Score
0	1.0
1	1.0
2	1.0
3	1.0
4	1.0
5	1.1
6	1.5
7	1.9
8	2.2
9	2.5
10	2.8
11	3.1
12	3.4
13	3.6
14	3.9
15	4.1
16	4.4
17	4.6
18	4.9
19	5.1
20	5.4
21	5.6
22	5.9
23	6.1
24	6.4
25	6.7
26	7.0
27	7.3
28	7.6
29	8.0
30	8.4
31	8.9
32	9.0
33	9.0
34	9.0
35	9.0

SECTION 2	
Number Correct	BMAT Score
0	1.0
1	1.0
2	1.0
3	1.3
4	1.8
5	2.2
6	2.6
7	2.9
8	3.2
9	3.5
10	3.7
11	4.0
12	4.2
13	4.5
14	4.7
15	4.9
16	5.2
17	5.4
18	5.6
19	5.9
20	6.2
21	6.5
22	6.8
23	7.2
24	7.7
25	8.3
26	9.0
27	9.0

N.B. These scores are for approximation purposes only. The scoring tables used for the BMAT vary slightly year to year, depending on student performance and the norming of the questions in each version of the test paper. To err on the side of caution, these scoring tables are among the toughest ever used on the BMAT. In most cases, a similar performance on the BMAT would result in a slightly higher score.

Test 6

BMAT
Section 1

Test ID Test 1 ○ Test 2 ○ Test 3 ○ Test 4 ○ Test 5 ○ Test 6 ●

Last Name

First Name

Date

Completely fill in the space for your intended answer choice

A B C D E
○ ○ ● ○ ○

1 A B C D E F ○ ○ ○ ○ ○ ○
2 A B C D E ○ ○ ○ ○ ○
3 A B C D E ○ ○ ○ ○ ○
4 A B C D E ○ ○ ○ ○ ○
5 A B C D E ○ ○ ○ ○ ○
6 A B C D E F G ○ ○ ○ ○ ○ ○ ○
7 A B C D E ○ ○ ○ ○ ○
8 A B C D E ○ ○ ○ ○ ○
9 A B C D E ○ ○ ○ ○ ○
10 A B C D E ○ ○ ○ ○ ○

11 A B C D E F ○ ○ ○ ○ ○ ○
12 A B C D E ○ ○ ○ ○ ○
13 A B C D E F G ○ ○ ○ ○ ○ ○ ○
14 A B C D E F ○ ○ ○ ○ ○ ○
15 A B C D E ○ ○ ○ ○ ○
16 A B C D E ○ ○ ○ ○ ○
17 A B C D E ○ ○ ○ ○ ○
18 A B C D E ○ ○ ○ ○ ○
19 A B C D ○ ○ ○ ○
20 A B C D E ○ ○ ○ ○ ○

21 A B C D ○ ○ ○ ○
22 A B C D E ○ ○ ○ ○ ○
23 A B C D E F ○ ○ ○ ○ ○ ○
24 A B C D E ○ ○ ○ ○ ○
25 A B C D ○ ○ ○ ○
26 A B C D E ○ ○ ○ ○ ○
27 A B C D E F ○ ○ ○ ○ ○ ○
28 A B C D E F ○ ○ ○ ○ ○ ○
29 A B C D E ○ ○ ○ ○ ○
30 A B C D E ○ ○ ○ ○ ○

31 A B C D E ○ ○ ○ ○ ○
32 A B C D ○ ○ ○ ○
33 A B C D ○ ○ ○ ○
34 A B C D E F G H ○ ○ ○ ○ ○ ○ ○ ○
35 A B C D ○ ○ ○ ○

BMAT
Section 2

KAPLAN
TEST PREP

	Test 1	Test 2	Test 3	Test 4	Test 5	Test 6
Test ID	○	○	○	○	○	●

Last Name

First Name

Date

Completely fill in the space for your intended answer choice

A B C D E
○ ○ ● ○ ○

1 A B C D E F G H
○ ○ ○ ○ ○ ○ ○ ○

2 A B C D E
○ ○ ○ ○ ○

3 A B C D E F
○ ○ ○ ○ ○ ○

4 A B C D E F
○ ○ ○ ○ ○ ○

5 A B C D
○ ○ ○ ○

6 A B C D E F
○ ○ ○ ○ ○ ○

7 A B C D E
○ ○ ○ ○ ○

8 A B C D E F
○ ○ ○ ○ ○ ○

9 A B C D E F G H
○ ○ ○ ○ ○ ○ ○ ○

10 A B C D E F G H
○ ○ ○ ○ ○ ○ ○ ○

11 A B C D E F
○ ○ ○ ○ ○ ○

12 A B C D E
○ ○ ○ ○ ○

13 A B C D E F
○ ○ ○ ○ ○ ○

14 A B C D E
○ ○ ○ ○ ○

15 A B C D E
○ ○ ○ ○ ○

16 A B C D E
○ ○ ○ ○ ○

17 A B C D
○ ○ ○ ○

18 A B C D E F
○ ○ ○ ○ ○ ○

19 A B C D E F
○ ○ ○ ○ ○ ○

20 A B C D E
○ ○ ○ ○ ○

21 A B C D E F
○ ○ ○ ○ ○ ○

22 A B C D E
○ ○ ○ ○ ○

23 A B C D E F G H
○ ○ ○ ○ ○ ○ ○ ○

24 A B C D E F G
○ ○ ○ ○ ○ ○ ○

25 A B C D E F G
○ ○ ○ ○ ○ ○ ○

26 A B C D E F G
○ ○ ○ ○ ○ ○ ○

27 A B C D E
○ ○ ○ ○ ○

K

BMAT is a registered trademark of Cambridge Assessment, which neither sponsors nor endorses this product.

BMAT
Section 3

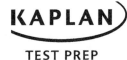

	Test 1	Test 2	Test 3	Test 4	Test 5	Test 6
Test ID	○	○	○	○	○	○

Last Name

First Name

Question answered

Your answer must be contained within this area.

BMAT is a registered trademark of Cambridge Assessment, which neither sponsors nor endorses this product.

243

BMAT SECTION 1: APTITUDE AND SKILLS (60 MINUTES)

You have 60 minutes to answer 35 questions. There are no penalties for incorrect answers, so you should attempt all questions.

Fill in your answers to each question on the answer sheet provided. Shade the circles corresponding to the answer choice(s) you have selected.

Avoid making stray marks on the paper. If you make a mistake, erase your answer completely and try again.

Calculators are **not** permitted.

1   The table below shows the cumulative number of apps downloaded from a leading app store by the end of each year indicated. For example, there were 11,000,000,000 more apps downloaded at the end of 2011 than at the end of 2010, meaning that this many apps were downloaded from the app store during 2011.

The table also shows the percentage of apps downloaded in each year that were only used once during the first six months after download.

Year	Cumulative number of apps downloaded (in billions)	Percentage of apps used only once during first 6 months
2010	7	26%
2011	18	26%
2012	35	22%
2013	60	22%
2014	85	20%
2015	100	25%

How many apps that were downloaded in 2013 were used more than once in the first six months after download?

A   5,500,000,000

B   11,700,000,000

C   13,200,000,000

D   19,500,000,000

E   20,500,000,000

F   46,800,000,000

2   At Trops Academy, a secondary school in Lancashire, students played hockey and football on the field during autumn term (September-December). In the spring and summer terms (January-June), they play these sports on the covered artificial grass pitch. During the academic year 2012-13, in the autumn term, players were reported to have had a total of 12 injuries, including 3 broken bones when they played on the field whereas in the spring and summer terms players were reported to have had 34 injuries, 9 of which were broken bones. It was concluded that playing on the field resulted in fewer injuries and was therefore safer than playing on the artificial grass; as a result, the school decided that all sports should be played on real grass throughout the year.

Which of the following, if true, would most help to weaken the argument above?

A   Looking back through the records, the same trend in injuries across the 2012-13 academic year was seen for the last eight academic years.

B   The following academic year saw a 15% decrease in the number of injuries sustained by sports players at Trops Academy.

C   Some sports, including tennis, cannot be played on the field when it is raining or when it has recently rained, as damp grass stops the ball from bouncing.

D   In the spring and summer term of 2013, football players didn't wear shin pads or mouth guards.

E   In the 2012-13 academic year, there were 3 hockey and football games during the autumn term and 45 games during the spring and summer terms.

3   Zoe designs websites for various companies, including the coding for the webpages as well as the graphics design. The price that she charges is based on the number of webpages on the site and whether the webpages are coded in HTML or Java. Her prices per webpage are summarised in the table below:

Number of webpages	HTML	Java
Up to 3	£90	£120
4 to 10	£75	£105
11 or more	£60	£80

Zoe also offers two types of graphics design services: still images (pics) and motion graphics. Still images cost £55 per pic and motion graphics cost £90 per page.

A company requests that Zoe design a website that includes 7 webpages. How much more would it cost for the webpages to be designed in Java with motion graphics on every page rather than in HTML with one pic per page?

A   £35

B   £195

C   £210

D   £385

E   £455

4   Researchers have recently examined 15-25 year olds' exam results to assess the effects of caffeine on memory. Caffeine is a psychoactive stimulant that has been shown to improve exam performance by increasing short-term memory recall. Students reported being able to retain more information for extended periods of time, after taking caffeine, and were less likely to experience the 'tip of the tongue' effect where they couldn't quite recall the answers. Thus, drinking a cup of coffee before your exam will make you perform better. Students must be aware, however, that they may experience caffeine withdrawal including headaches and fatigue.

What is the central argument upon which the argument above depends?

A   Improving memory recall will improve exam performance.

B   Coffee is a source of caffeine.

C   Caffeine withdrawal could have a negative impact on students' performance in exams.

D   Psychoactive stimulants improve exam performance.

E   Drinking coffee can increase your test score.

5   Alicia, Lily, Chloe, Freya and Hannah make up the girl group Saffron Nights. Their surnames are Davies, Hall, Swain, Wood and Young, but my friend is struggling to recall which surname goes with which first name.

I tell my friend that no letter appears more than twice in each girl's full names (first name plus surname) and that each girl's first name contains a different number of letters than her surname.

What is Chloe's surname?

A   Davies

B   Hall

C   Swain

D   Wood

E   Young

6   The United Kingdom has been in a recession since 2008. In the years since there have been several changes across all industries to the UK workforce. In the current socioeconomic climate, there is a vicious cycle emerging with employers expecting increasingly more from their employees and, as a result, employees putting in increasingly longer hours at work, above and beyond their contracted hours, to the detriment of their general wellbeing and work/life balance. Working hours should therefore be legally reduced from 40 hours per week to 25 hours per week. Employees work more efficiently in short bursts meaning the same amount of work could be achieved in this shorter time frame and a higher hourly rate would ensure no employee misses out financially.

Which of the following indicate flaws in the argument above?

1   Limiting working hours without reducing workloads would make employees even more overworked.

2   Most employees in the UK worked more than 40 hours per week prior to the start of the recession in 2008.

3   Reducing working hours would allow employees to spend more time pursuing leisure and social activities.

A   1 only

B   2 only

C   3 only

D   1 and 2

E   1 and 3

F   2 and 3

G   1, 2 and 3

7   A group of friends are attending a charity dinner, where they have all been given a raffle ticket numbered from 1 to 12. The friends are to be seated at the same round table based on the number on their raffle ticket, which will determine their seats in order to meet a list of criteria given to them by the charity. A partial seating plan is shown below:

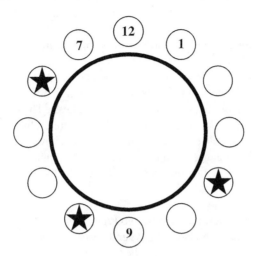

The charity requires that the friends arrange themselves in groups of four, known as 'squares'. Each square will consist of four seats that would form a square, if lines were drawn from each seat in the square to the nearest seats (to its left or right) that are also part of the same square. For example, the three seats marked with stars form a square with the seat at the upper-right of the table, which must be taken by the friend holding ticket number 1 (which is thereby known as 'seat 1').

The charity further requires that the friends in each square are seated so that the corners of each square increase in value as you go around the table the long way from seat 1 to seat 12.

Finally, the charity requires that the total sum of the ticket numbers in one of the squares equals the total sum of the ticket numbers in another square; the sum of the ticket numbers of the third square is more than the total sum of the ticket numbers of these two squares combined.

What will be the ticket number of the friend sitting in the seat next to seat 7 that is marked with a star?

A   4

B   5

C   6

D   10

E   11

Questions 8 to 11 refer to the following information:

Global warming, with its resulting impact on the weather and rising sea levels, is one of the greatest challenges for today's society. Since the Industrial Revolution, the emission of greenhouse gases has risen significantly with detrimental effects on the environment. There are several gases responsible for this enhanced greenhouse effect, with varying potencies. Methane is the most potent, causing four times the amount of damage per gram than carbon dioxide and nitrous oxide. Activists claim that we must take action, sooner rather than later, before it is too late to reverse the effects. So it is clear; we must reduce carbon dioxide emissions in the UK.

One of the ways the UK government is tackling the issue is through the planting of trees. Trees produce a small amount of carbon dioxide through a process called respiration however; they also use carbon dioxide and turn it into oxygen through a process known as photosynthesis. Therefore, any net oxygen output can also be thought of as the amount of carbon dioxide absorbed by the tree. This initiative is paid for through public funding and it is important to be able to collect valuable data to show the effectiveness of the programme. If the programme is shown to be effective, then more trees will be planted at sites across the UK, with a goal of reducing the UK's net carbon dioxide output and reducing the harmful effects of greenhouse gases on our climate and sea levels.

In a small patch of woodland in North Somerset, two types of trees were planted three years ago. The aim was to find out which species had a higher net oxygen output (carbon dioxide absorption) and to observe how these outputs change over time, as trees mature. The tables below indicate the oxygen and carbon dioxide production of these two trees during this trial period.

Oxygen Production

	2013	2014	2015
English Oak	521 g	543 g	572 g
Rosewood	274 g	314 g	295 g

Carbon Dioxide Production

	2013	2014	2015
English Oak	210 g	211 g	196 g
Rosewood	111 g	153 g	131 g

8   What was the net production of oxygen by both trees over the three years of the trial period?

   A   1012 g

   B   1287 g

   C   1507 g

   D   1910 g

   E   2519 g

9   By how much did the net oxygen production of the English oak tree increase from 2013 to 2014?

    A   2.25%

    B   3.33%

    C   5.15%

    D   6.33%

    E   6.75%

10   Which of the following, if true, would be the most likely to weaken the effectiveness of the tree planting scheme?

    A   Most nitrous oxide is emitted into the atmosphere during the manufacture and use of agricultural fertilisers.

    B   The impact of carbon dioxide on the temperature and sea levels, as compared to that of other greenhouse gases, is negligible.

    C   Methane has a less potent effect on the temperature and sea levels than carbon dioxide.

    D   Carbon dioxide is the most prevalent of all gases that contribute to the greenhouse effect.

    E   The impact of greenhouse gases on our quality of life is less potent now than it was during the Industrial Revolution.

11   What was the ratio of oxygen to carbon dioxide output for the rosewood tree in 2015?

    A   3 : 4

    B   4 : 3

    C   5 : 3

    D   9 : 4

    E   5 : 2

    F   7 : 2

12   Road humps cost more lives than they save. This is because they obstruct the passage of ambulances, increasing the time it takes for medical help to reach seriously ill or injured patients, as well as making it impossible for paramedics to provide lifesaving treatment to patients when on the move. 90% of victims survive if treated within 2 minutes, but it falls to 10% if treatment is delayed for 6 minutes. On a typical route in London, ambulances are thought to be slowed by, on average, four minutes per journey. Clearly, road humps should be eliminated in London.

What role does the following statement play in the above argument?

'Road humps cost more lives than they save'

A   It introduces information which makes the argument's conclusion more likely to be true.

B   It states the main point of the argument.

C   It concedes a point that would seem to undermine the argument's conclusion.

D   It explains that although road safety methods are not fool-proof, they are largely beneficial.

E   It summarises the justification for the argument's conclusion.

13   My flatmate has two 24-hour digital watches. One of them is normally 15 minutes slow and the other is normally 6 minutes slow. I don't understand why my flatmate keeps them like this, but I do know that since the most recent time change, my flatmate forgot to put the watch that it was 6 minutes slow forward by an hour, so it is now 1 hour and 6 minutes slow. At the same time, my flatmate mistakenly put the other watch forward by two hours, so it is now 45 minutes fast.

As a result, it means that once every 24 hours, for three minutes in a row, the two watches display eight completely different digits each minute.

Which of the following times appears on one of the watches during one of the three minutes in a row when all eight digits are different?

A   17:34

B   18:45

C   18:54

D   19:37

E   20:46

F   23:47

G   23:56

14 My favourite flavour of jam at the local supermarket is damson, which is normally sold in three jar sizes, as follows:

$$
\begin{array}{lcl}
\text{small} & - & 150\ \text{g} \\
\text{medium} & - & 250\ \text{g} \\
\text{large} & - & 500\ \text{g}
\end{array}
$$

At the moment, there is a special offer at the supermarket, so that all three jars contain 30% extra jam for the normal price and, in addition, anyone who buys a large jar will be given a small jar at no extra charge.

If I buy a large jar of jam during the special offer, what is the total additional percentage of jam that I will take home, compared to buying a large jar purchased prior to the special offer?

A   43%

B   46%

C   50%

D   59%

E   69%

F   77%

15 Married couples should not be so eager to rush into couples' counselling in an attempt to strengthen their relationship. Couples' therapy is likely to put a strain on relationships, as couples often compete for the therapist's attention, in order to get the therapist on 'their side,' thereby increasing the rift between partners. Statistics show that the majority of couples who eventually file for a divorce will go to at least one couples therapy session before they separate.

Which of the following, if true, would be the most likely to weaken the above argument?

A   Many couples who do not attend a couple's therapy session also break up.

B   Individuals who regularly attend therapy sessions are calmer and more considerate than individuals who do not.

C   Married couples only attend couples therapy when they feel their relationship is already at risk.

D   Married couples who do not attend couples therapy are often happier than those who do.

E   Some couples who attend couples therapy do not get a divorce.

16   The floor of my kitchen is covered with 49 tiles to form a 7 by 7 square. Each tile consists of a white 2 by 2 grid, with one or more of the quadrants shaded black. Some of the tiles may have black quadrants that do not line up exactly with the 2 by 2 grid; for example, they may have a black quadrant in the centre of the tile, or centred along one side.

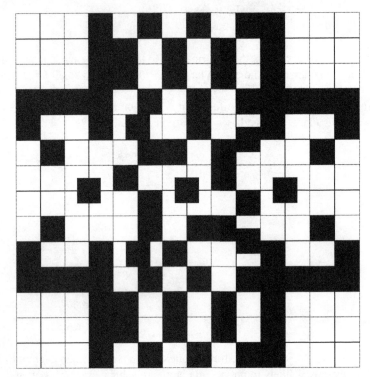

How many distinct types of tiles are there in my floor?

A   7

B   8

C   9

D   10

E   11

17   The number of nurses being trained in Britain has fallen by 20% in recent years. As such, for the next three years Britain will solve this issue by offering 5,000 visas to overseas nurses, allowing them to come and work in Britain. Whether there are less nurses because the British population as a whole no longer has the same interest in nursing, whether it is now too expensive to train to become a nurse in Britain, or whether it is simply that less courses are now offered in Britain to nurses, the only answer to the shortage is to import nurses from overseas.

Which of the following best describes the central assumption of the argument above?

A   It is not possible for Britain to create more nursing courses, reduce the cost of training to be a nurse or revive interest in nursing.

B   It is possible that the current nursing shortage is due to reasons other than the expense and availability of nursing courses.

C   In Britain, it is currently too difficult to train to be a nurse.

D   Nurses are trained to a higher quality overseas.

E   Importing nurses will permanently solve the shortage of nurses in Britain.

18   Green, white, oolong and black tea are all made from the leaves of the same plant, *camellia sinensis*. The exposure, or level of oxidation of the tea leaves, determines what type of tea the leaves will become. White tea tends to contain the least amount of caffeine, whereas black tea typically contains the most caffeine, although the caffeine levels can also vary due to how the tea is prepared, the amount of tea used, the water temperature and the brewing time. As such, a cup of black tea can contain from 16 mg of caffeine to in excess of 40 mg. The many variables involved in tea brewing is one of the reasons tea remains to be such a popular beverage

Which **one** of the following can be safely inferred from the above argument?

A   A tea will always contain more caffeine if more leaves are used.

B   Oolong tea and black tea are exposed to different levels of oxidation during production.

C   Black tea should taste stronger than green tea.

D   White tea must contain less than 16 mg of caffeine.

E   Green tea must contain less than 40 mg of caffeine.

Questions 19 to 22 refer to the following information:

A recent study has revealed a sharp rise in the use of antidepressants (ATD) to treat patients who are children, despite the fact that the NHS advises against prescribing ATD to patients aged under 18. The study looked at the rates of ATD use in five countries – the UK, the US, the Netherlands, Denmark and Germany – in 2005 and 2012. The research indicated that the US had the highest use of ATD in children aged 19 and under (1.6% of those aged 5 to 19), followed by the UK (1.1% of the same age group), Denmark (1.0%), the Netherlands (0.6%) and Germany (0.5%). By comparison, only 0.7% of children the same ages in the UK were prescribed ATD in 2005, reflecting a rise of over 50%. (ATD are never prescribed to children under the age of 5, so children aged 0–4 are not included in the study's statistics.)

The study considers anyone aged 19 and under to be a child, since these countries gather population statistics in 5-year brackets. For example, here are the brackets for the UK's child population in 2012:

Aged 0–4:	3,996,400
Aged 5–9:	3,640,999
Aged 10–14:	3,576,365
Aged 15–19:	3,926,550

The UK population was 63,700,000 in 2012, and a total of 4 million people in the UK of all ages were taking ATD in that year. There are two main categories of ATD: selective serotonin reuptake inhibitors (SSRI), such as Prozac and Seroxat, which work by increasing serotonin levels in the brain, and tricyclic antidepressants (TCA), such as Tryptizol and Allegron, which block the effects of serotonin and norepinephrine in the brain. TCA are a much older class of ATD, dating to the 1950s, and they have generally fallen out of favour in the global medical community, having been displaced by SSRI. However, data from the study determined that 19.5% of all ATD prescribed in the UK in 2012 were TCA, with the rest consisting of SSRI. Furthermore, the data seem to suggest that TCA are more commonly given to older patients in the UK: 90% of ATD prescribed to teenagers aged 15 to 19 in the UK in 2012 were SSRI.

What is driving the rise in ATD used to treat children in the UK? It is commonly accepted that pressures on other NHS services, such as therapy, that would otherwise be used to treat depression in children are a factor. Indeed, the NHS only suggests that ATD be used to treat children in combination with 'talk therapy' or following an attempt at talk therapy, due to the risk of side effects from taking ATD. There is another explanation to consider: the normalisation of 'pill-a-day' culture, as a significant proportion of the population must now take a pill at least once a day for the rest of their lives, for any number of chronic conditions. This leads to the mindset that if you have a problem, all you need to do is pop a pill and it will sort you out. This would go some way to explaining why so many parents are so accepting of ATD prescriptions in younger children. For example, in the UK, the greatest rise in ATD use from 2005 to 2012 was among children aged 10–14.

19   How many people in the UK aged 19 and under were prescribed antidepressants in 2012?

A   117,085

B   122,583

C   139,299

D   142,630

20   Which of the following, if true, would be the most likely to strengthen the argument about 'pill-a-day' culture as a factor in increased rates of antidepressant use among children in the UK?

A   A majority of the children prescribed antidepressants in the UK in 2012 had at least one parent who took a daily prescription for a long-term medical condition.

B   Most adults in the UK in 2012 took a pill prescribed by a doctor at least once a day.

C   Fewer parents of UK children who were prescribed antidepressants in 2012 took a pill at least once a day, as compared to parents of UK children who were prescribed antidepressants in 2005.

D   Fewer parents in the UK took a daily antidepressant in 2012, as compared to the same group in 2005.

E   More parents of children in the UK who were prescribed antidepressants in 2012 were also prescribed antidepressants themselves than parents of children in the US who were prescribed antidepressants in that same year.

21   What proportion of the UK population aged 5 and older were taking selective serotonin reuptake inhibitors or tricyclic antidepressants in 2012?

A   5.9%

B   6.2%

C   6.7%

D   7.2%

Question 22 refers to the previous information as well as the following additional information:

The table below includes the percentages of UK children in the age brackets indicated that were prescribed antidepressants in 2005 and 2012.

	2005	2012
Aged 10–14	0.7%	1.2%
Aged 15–19	1.5%	1.8%

22   How many teenagers in the UK aged 15 to 19 were prescribed selective serotonin reuptake inhibitors in 2012?

A   42,407

B   48,281

C   56,896

D   57,937

E   63,610

23   My brother has four children: Louis, Jade, Kieran and Molly. Their birthdays (outside of leap years) fall on the 83rd, 238th, 283rd and 328th days of the year, respectively.

Which two of my brother's children have their birthdays on the same day of the week as each other (except in leap years)?

A   Jade and Kieran

B   Jade and Louis

C   Jade and Molly

D   Kieran and Louis

E   Kieran and Molly

F   Louis and Molly

24   Up until as late as 1934, it wasn't necessary to have a driving license in order to drive. Since then, it has been made illegal to drink alcohol and drive, or to use a phone while driving, as these activities decrease the driver's concentration on the road, increasing the likelihood of a road traffic accident. Most recently, road safety officials are looking into the dangers of live streaming from a mobile phone while driving. It is clear that technology has led to an unprecedented increase in risks to road safety that the law is struggling to keep up with.

Which of the following, if true, would help to weaken the above argument the most?

A   More road fatalities are caused by drivers and passengers not wearing seat belts than by drivers texting while driving.

B   In the UK, the number of drivers who choose to live stream while driving is very small.

C   Road safety officials have looked into the effects of other actions performed while driving, and ultimately decided that such actions did not pose a risk.

D   Some people are able to use their mobile phones while driving with minimal loss of concentration.

E   Recent changes to driving laws, such as child car seat restrictions and the new offence of 'drug driving' (driving while under the influence of illegal drugs), are not linked to any technology used while driving.

25 The draw for the qualifying round of the Audubon Cup has just taken place.

There are eight teams competing in Group A of the qualifying round of the Audubon Cup, and each of these teams was represented by a number from 1 to 8, as follows:

1   Bluebirds
2   Cranes
3   Eagles
4   Herons
5   Kestrels
6   Ospreys
7   Swans
8   Teals

To determine the order of play, eight balls (also numbered from 1 to 8) were drawn from a tombola, one by one. The first teams corresponding to the numbers on the first two balls drawn will play each other in the qualifying round, as will the third and fourth teams, the fifth and sixth teams, and the final two teams.

Whilst the balls were selected at random, there was always a difference of 4 or less between the numbers on one ball and the next ball, and the balls continued to alternate between odd and even numbers throughout the draw.

The first ball drawn was number 7 (Swans) and the final ball drawn was number 6 (Ospreys).

Which of the following statements must be true regarding the teams competing in Group A of the qualifying round of the Audubon Cup?

A   The Eagles were selected 5th in the draw and will play either the Cranes or the Herons.

B   The Herons were selected 2nd in the draw and will play the Swans.

C   The Kestrels were selected 3rd in the draw and will play either the Cranes or the Herons.

D   The Teals were selected 4th in the draw and will play the Kestrels.

26 In England, the majority of us purchase readymade meals on a weekly, if not daily, basis. The government is committed to helping people to cook and assemble more meals for themselves in a cost efficient manner. We need to understand that if we want to know what our food is made up of, the only way to ensure that we avoid any unhealthy or otherwise disagreeable ingredients is to make all of our meals from scratch.

Which of the following is the best statement of the central assumption in the argument above?

A   The longer it takes to create a meal, the better the quality of the meal.

B   Cooking from scratch is only permissible if the cost of the component parts is cheaper than the equivalent readymade meal.

C   Readymade meals should be avoided as they take less of an effort to make.

D   Readymade meals could contain harmful or unpleasant ingredients.

E   As long as all of the ingredients are included, it is permissible for us to cook our own meals as opposed to buying food readymade.

27 Noah had 180 Wazzits that he wanted to sell, so he hired a stall on a nearby weekend street market.

On the Saturday, the Wazzits were priced at £24 each, and Noah was surprised that he sold less than 20% of them.

On the Sunday, Noah sold exactly three times as many Wazzits, and he took £696 more than he did on the Saturday. As a result, at the end of the weekend, Noah had less than 40% of his original stock remaining.

How many Wazzits did Noah sell on Saturday and Sunday?

A   87

B   96

C   105

D   110

E   116

F   121

28 The four digits of the PIN for my debit card are all different digits (from zero to nine). When the digits are written as words, they are in alphabetical order (from left to right), and exactly two of digits contain the same number of letters; these two digits are not adjacent to each other (from left to right) in my PIN. Furthermore, the total number of letters is the same as the numerical sum of the digits in my PIN.

One of the digits in my PIN is nine.

Which digits must appear adjacent to each other (from left to right) in my PIN?

A   2 and 0

B   3 and 2

C   6 and 7

D   7 and 2

E   8 and 9

F   9 and 6

29   Currently, it is illegal for anyone to sell rhino horns in South Africa, due to the fact that most rhino horns are obtained illicitly, by poachers. Poachers will often kill rhinos in order to harvest their horns, and are threatening the already endangered rhino population in South Africa. It is possible for rhino owners to harvest their animals' horns without killing them. Allowing rhino owners to then sell these horns would offer the owners an incentive to carry out the costly operation. If rhino owners were legally allowed to sell their rhinos' horns, it would dramatically improve their rhinos' chances of survival.

The argument above depends upon which of the following assumptions?

A   Removing rhinos' horns increases their overall health.

B   Poachers would stop attempting to sell rhino horn illegally if rhino owners were allowed to sell rhino horn legally.

C   Rhinos without horns are unlikely to be targeted by poachers.

D   When rhino horns are not harvested and sold, money is wasted.

E   Without horns, rhinos would be better able to defend themselves against poachers.

30   On a day trip to a local lake, four friends want to go for a ride in a pedalo. (A pedalo is a boat powered by pushing pedals with the feet, somewhat similar to riding a bicycle.)

The friends have the option of hiring three different capacities of pedalo:

Individual: £30/hour   Paired: £24/hour   Group: £36/hour
(1 person)   (2 people)   (2 to 4 people)

Each pedalo must be hired for a minimum of two hours. The friends want to ride in at least two different pedalos.

Special offers:
15% discount for 3 or more pedalos hired together
10% discount for 2 pedalos hired together

One of the friends has a voucher for £25 which can be used once to hire a group pedalo. The voucher is applied after any special offers.

What is the cheapest option?

A   Four individual pedalos

B   Two paired pedalos

C   One group pedalo and one paired pedalo

D   One group pedalo and one individual pedalo

E   One paired pedalo and two individual pedalos

31 One of the activities at a recent village fete was 'Balloon Car,' in which you buy a ticket allowing you to guess the number of balloons inside a 2-door car. The entirety of the inside of the car, including the boot, was packed full of standard-sized balloons that are fully inflated. Each ticket entitles you to guess a number of balloons, and the prizes are awarded according to how close each guess came to the exact number. Each number could be guessed only once.

Prize	Guess	Winner
1st	307	Kian
2nd	296	Tess
3rd	293	Huw
4th	313	Lakeisha
5th	314	George
6th	285	Amira

How many balloons were inside the car?

A   299

B   300

C   301

D   302

E   303

Questions 32 to 35 refer to the following information:

Global Airlines is offering a special 'round-the-world' fare of £3570, which allows for up to 16 flights in a period of up to a year. Alternately, you could book individual flights, starting and ending in London, as indicated in the table below. All prices (including the special fare) are given in British pounds. All flight times are based on travel in the summer, when the time in London is GMT +1.

Flight	Departure time	Time difference	Flight length	Distance (in air miles)	Price
London → Rio	12:20	−4	11 h, 40 min	5800	£650
Rio → San Francisco	21:10	−4	16 h, 20 min	6700	£380
San Francisco → Sydney	23:25	+17	14 h, 35 min	7400	£800
Sydney → Bangkok	09:50	−3	9 h, 50 min	4700	£520
Bangkok → Nairobi	00:35	−4	8 h, 50 min	4500	£900
Nairobi → London	23:20	−2	8 h, 55 min	4200	£700

All flights are non-stop, except for the flight from Rio to San Francisco, which requires you to change planes in Houston, with a layover of 1 hr, 50 min. This layover is included in the overall flight time for the journey from Rio to San Francisco.

You cross the International Date Line when flying from San Francisco to Sydney. For example, when it is 23:54 Sunday in San Francisco, it is 16:54 Monday (17 hours later) in Sydney.

In order to visit all seven continents, there is the option of a side trip to Antarctica, which would come after arrival in Rio but before departure to San Francisco. The airfare from Rio to the cruise port (Punta Arenas, Chile) and the price of the cruise to Antarctica (which depends on the type of cabin) would be additional costs:

Flights from Rio to Punta Arenas (via Santiago): 2500 air miles each way; return airfare £270

Cruise to Antarctica, starting/ending in Punta Arenas (9 days; 6100 total miles): £3,200 in a shared cabin; £5,400 in a private cabin

Time zones: The time in Santiago is the same as Rio (GMT −3); the time in Antarctica is 15 hours ahead of Santiago (GMT +12). Antarctic time is based on the time at the South Pole, which is always 12 hours ahead of GMT.

32   How much would you save by booking the special fare, instead of the individual flights listed, if you decide not to go on the side trip to Antarctica?

A   8.8%

B   9.6%

C   10.6%

D   11.9%

33 Suppose that you wanted to travel around the world as quickly as possible, starting and ending in London, using only the flights listed and opting out of the side trip to Antarctica. Suppose as well that you must allow at least 90 minutes between flights, in order to re-check bags, clear security, and so forth.

If you departed London for Rio on a Monday, when is the earliest you could arrive back in London on the flight from Nairobi (assuming all flights arrive and depart at the scheduled times)?

A Saturday morning

B Saturday evening

C Sunday morning

D the following Monday morning

34 Which of the following is a safe inference to draw from the data regarding Antarctica?

1 Adding the Antarctic cruise and related flights increases the overall mileage for the round-the-world trip by one-third.

2 Adding the Antarctic cruise and related flights more than doubles the overall travel cost of the round-the-world fare.

3 When it is 11 a.m. at the South Pole, it is 9 a.m. the same day in Sydney.

4 When it is 11 a.m. at the South Pole, it is 9 p.m. the previous day in Santiago.

A 2 only

B 3 only

C 1 and 2

D 1 and 3

E 1, 2 and 3

F 1, 2 and 4

G 1, 3 and 4

H 2, 3 and 4

35 If the air mileage from Rio to Houston is 5,031 miles, then the flight from Houston to San Francisco is what percentage of the journey from Rio to San Francisco?

A 25%

B 30%

C 75%

D 80%

BMAT SECTION 2: SCIENTIFIC KNOWLEDGE AND APPLICATIONS (30 MINUTES)

You have 30 minutes to answer 27 questions. There are no penalties for incorrect answers, so you should attempt all questions.

Fill in your answers to each question on the answer sheet provided. Shade the circles corresponding to the answer choice(s) you have selected.

Avoid making stray marks on the paper. If you make a mistake, erase your answer completely and try again.

Calculators are **not** permitted.

1   The following statements relate to enzymes:

    1   Enzymes only function properly at high temperatures.

    2   Enzymes accelerate chemical reactions that are helpful to the body.

    3   Enzymes consist of amino acids, which are folded into unique shapes that allow the enzyme to function.

    4   Enzymes function as a 'key' which fits into a particular substrate (the 'lock') in the 'lock and key' model.

Which statements are correct?

    A   1 and 2

    B   2 and 3

    C   3 and 4

    D   1, 2 and 3

    E   1, 2 and 4

    F   1, 3 and 4

    G   2, 3 and 4

    H   All

2   An organic compound is found to contain 6 parts of carbon, 1 part of hydrogen and 8 parts of oxygen by mass. 18 g of a gaseous sample of the compound would have a volume of 4.8 dm^3 at room temperature and standard pressure. (A_r: H = 1; C = 12; O = 16)
(1 mole of any gas occupies 24 dm^3 at room temperature and pressure)

Which of the following is the molecular formula for this compound?

    A CH_6O

    B C_2HO_2

    C $C_3H_6O_3$

    D $C_3H_{10}O_3$

    E C_4HO_4

3   A builder calculates that he transferred 40 watts of power in carrying an armchair with a mass of 30 kg a total distance of 200 metres from a house into a removals van, accelerating at a rate of 2 m/s^2.

How long was the builder carrying the armchair?

    A   3 minutes

    B   5 minutes

    C   6 minutes

    D   10 minutes

    E   12 minutes

    F   15 minutes

4   If you look at a clock and the time is 2:30, with the hour hand equidistant between the 2 and the 3, what is the angle between the hour and the minute hands on the clock?

    A   75°

    B   90°

    C   100°

    D   105°

    E   120°

    F   135°

5   The family tree below is meant to show the inheritance of polydactyly, a genetic disorder in which babies are born with extra fingers or toes. However, there are errors in some of the individuals, as it is not possible for only the two individuals indicated (individual 2 and individual 7) to have polydactyly, while no one else in the family tree does.

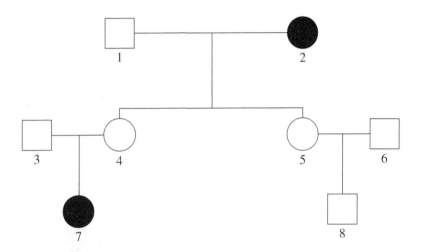

If at least one individual is correctly indicated as having polydactyly and at least two individuals are incorrectly identified as not having polydactyly, then which of the following must be true?

    A   At least one individual in the second generation has polydactyly.

    B   At least one of individual 7's parents has polydactyly.

    C   Both individuals in the first generation have polydactyly.

    D   Both of individual 7's parents have polydactyly.

Cyclohexene, C_6H_{10} is drawn as:

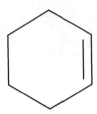

6   What is the total number of carbon atoms in the molecule indicated in the diagram below?

O

$CH3$

$C2H6$

$CH3$

A   22

B   24

C   25

D   26

E   33

F   38

7   What is the total resistance in the circuit shown below, if $r = 1\ \Omega$?

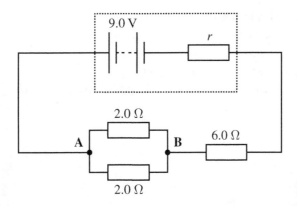

A $7\ \Omega$

B $8\ \Omega$

C $9\ \Omega$

D $11\ \Omega$

E $12\ \Omega$

8   The right-angled triangle shown in the diagram has a hypotenuse measuring $10\sqrt{2}$ cm and a vertical side measuring $4\sqrt{5}$ cm.

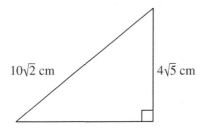

Calculate the area of the triangle.

A $2\sqrt{30}$

B $6\sqrt{7}$

C $7\sqrt{10}$

D $10\sqrt{7}$

E $20\sqrt{6}$

F $20\sqrt{10}$

9   The following statements relate to the control of blood glucose:

1   The pancreas withholds insulin when blood sugar levels are high.
2   Insulin causes glucose in the blood to move into cells.
3   The liver removes excess glucose when blood sugar levels are high.
4   Insulin is released when blood sugar levels are low.
5   You can remove some excess glucose from the blood by exercising vigorously.

Which statements are correct?

A   1, 2 and 3

B   1, 2 and 4

C   1, 3 and 5

D   1, 4 and 5

E   2, 3 and 4

F   2, 3 and 5

G   2, 4 and 5

H   3, 4 and 5

10   Which of the following atoms and ions contain exactly 24 electrons?

1   **20, 40** Ca
2   **11, 22** Na
3   **20, 40** Ca3$^-$
4   **22, 48** Ti2$^-$
5   **28, 58** Ni4$^+$

A   1 only

B   2 only

C   2 and 3 only

D   2 and 4 only

E   2 and 5 only

F   3 and 4 only

G   3 and 5 only

H   4 and 5 only

11 A research group discover a radioactive source. They place a detector close to the radioactive source and take 7 readings over a space of 7 minutes. They then place a sheet of paper between the detector and the source and then observe again the counts over 7 minutes. They then repeat this again, once by replacing the paper with aluminium and then with lead. Their results are shown below:

Reading	Nothing	Paper	Aluminium	Lead
1	98	76	75	0
2	102	74	77	0
3	99	77	79	1
4	100	75	73	0
5	103	78	76	0
6	101	77	74	1
7	102	76	78	0

What types of radiation is being given off by the source?

A α only

B β only

C γ only

D α and β

E α and γ

F β and γ

12 Given that $m = \sqrt{n}$, that m and n are both integers, and that $m^x + n^y = (mn)^z$, express z in terms of x and y.

A $z = \dfrac{1}{3}x + y$

B $z = \dfrac{x - 2y}{3}$

C $z = x + 2y$

D $z = \dfrac{x + 2y}{3}$

E $z = x - 2y$

13   Which of the following correctly describes what happens when body temperature drops in a human?

	muscles	arterioles (small arteries)	temperature change detected by	hair erector muscles
A	contract	constrict	hypothalamus	contract
B	contract	dilate	hypothalamus	contract
C	relax	constrict	hypothalamus	relax
D	relax	dilate	pituitary gland	relax
E	contract	constrict	pituitary gland	relax
F	relax	dilate	pituitary gland	contract

14   Bromobutane (C_4H_9Br) reacts with sodium hydroxide to produce butanol (C_4H_9OH) and sodium bromide, as indicated in the reaction equation below.

$C_4H_9Br + NaHO \rightarrow C_4H_9OH + NaBr$

(A_r: H = 1; C = 12; O = 16; Na = 23; Br = 80)

How much butanol will be produced if 274 g of bromobutane reacts with excess sodium hydroxide and the reaction has a 100% yield?

A   103 g

B   148 g

C   174 g

D   206 g

E   296 g

15   What acceleration is achieved if an object with a mass of 8 kg is exerted with a force of double its weight?

(Assume there is no drag and that $g = 10$ N/kg.)

A 2 m/s^2

B 5 m/s^2

C 10 m/s^2

D 20 m/s^2

E 40 m/s^2

16 Simplify:

$$(x^2+9)\left(\frac{x+3}{x^4-81}\right)$$

A $\dfrac{1}{x-3}$

B x^2-9

C $\dfrac{1}{x+3}$

D $x-3$

E $\dfrac{1}{x^2-9}$

17 The diagram below represents blood flow through a kidney dialysis machine. The machine is used for patients with advanced kidney disease. Toxins diffuse across membranes within the dialysis machine.

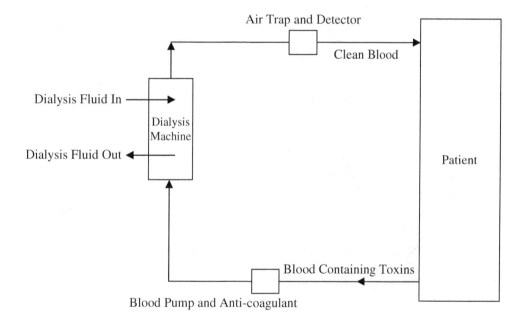

Which answer choice explains why toxins leave the patient's blood in the dialysis machine?

	Concentration of:			
	Toxin in dialysis fluid leaving machine	Toxin in dialysis fluid entering machine	Toxin in blood entering the patient	Toxin in blood leaving the patient
A	high	high	low	high
B	low	low	high	high
C	high	low	low	high
D	low	high	high	low

18   Which of the following are redox reactions?

1    $Zn + Cu^{2+} + SO_4^{2-} \rightarrow Cu + Zn^{2+} + SO_4^{2-}$
2    $Na_2CO_3 + SiO_2 \rightarrow Na_2SiO_3 + CO_2$
3    $HCl + KOH \rightarrow KCl + H_2O$
4    $Cl_2 + 2Fe^{2+} \rightarrow 2Cl^- + 2Fe^{3+}$

A   1 and 2 only

B   1 and 3 only

C   1 and 4 only

D   2 and 3 only

E   2 and 4 only

F   3 and 4 only

19   The displacement/time graph below represents a wave of wavelength of 4.5 cm.

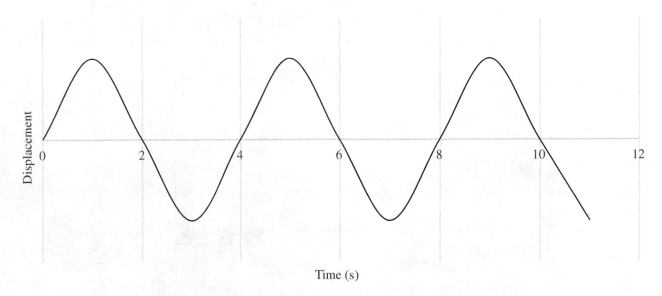

Time (s)

What is the speed of the wave?

A   0.57 cm/s

B   1.13 cm/s

C   2.25 cm/s

D   3.37 cm/s

E   4.50 cm/s

F   6.23 cm/s

20   A large equilateral triangle is formed by three smaller equilateral triangles (each with sides of length s) and three parallelograms.

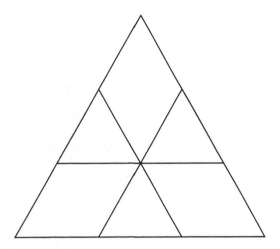

What is the area of the large equilateral triangle?

A $\left(\dfrac{3\sqrt{3}}{2}\right)s^2$

B $\left(\dfrac{9\sqrt{3}}{4}\right)s^2$

C $(3\sqrt{3})\,s^2$

D $(6\sqrt{3})\,s^2$

E $(12\sqrt{3})\,s^2$

21   The following statements relate to the nuclear division of cells:

1   Mitosis results in genetic variation within a species.
2   Meiosis if not correctly regulated can cause tumours.
3   Mitosis results in the production of diploid cells.
4   Mitosis is essential for the growth and maintenance of an organism.
5   Meiosis results in the production of haploid cells.

Which statements are correct?

A   1, 2 and 3

B   1, 2 and 4

C   1, 3 and 4

D   2, 3 and 4

E   2, 4 and 5

F   3, 4 and 5

22   A metal (referred to by the variable **Y**) is in Group 1 of the periodic table. A non-metal (referred to by the variable **Z**) is in Group 16 of the periodic table. They react to form a compound. What is the formula of the compound?

    A   **YZ**

    B $\mathbf{YZ_2}$

    C $\mathbf{Y_2Z}$

    D $\mathbf{Y_2Z_3}$

    E $\mathbf{Y_3Z_2}$

23   Below are four statements about electromagnetic radiation:

    1   Infrared radiation has the highest frequency of all electromagnetic waves.

    2   At identical amplitudes, microwaves have the lowest energy of all electromagnetic waves.

    3   Gamma radiation can cause genetic mutations that can lead to cancer.

    4   The wavelength of electromagnetic waves is inversely proportional to their frequency.

Which statements are correct?

    A   2 only

    B   3 only

    C   1 and 2 only

    D   1 and 3 only

    E   1 and 4 only

    F   2 and 3 only

    G   2 and 4 only

    H   3 and 4 only

24   A test has been developed to indicate a mental health condition. The test is not 100% accurate and can give false results. To test the reliability of the test, 2000 members of the population took the test and the results are shown in the tree diagram.

M = has the condition
M* = does not have the condition
P = tests positive for the condition
P* = tests negative for the condition

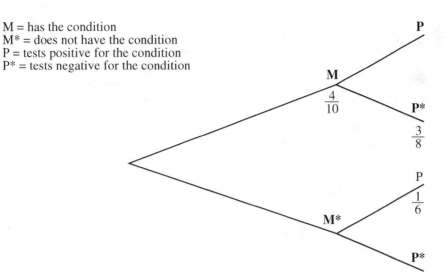

A person is selected at random from these 2000 people and tests negative for the condition. What is the probability that this person does not the condition?

A $\dfrac{3}{10}$

B $\dfrac{19}{60}$

C $\dfrac{2}{5}$

D $\dfrac{1}{2}$

E $\dfrac{5}{8}$

F $\dfrac{11}{16}$

G $\dfrac{4}{5}$

25   Graphite is formed when carbon atoms are linked together with three covalent bonds. The diagram shows a simplified structure of graphite.

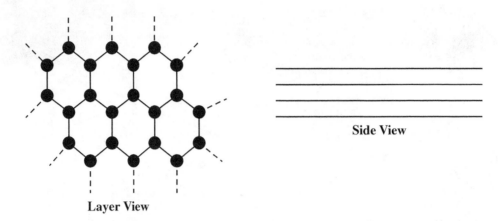

Considering its structure, which of the properties below could be predicted about graphite?

1   It conducts heat.
2   It has strong intermolecular forces between the layers.
3   It has a high melting point.

A   1 only

B   2 only

C   3 only

D   1 and 2 only

E   1 and 3 only

F   2 and 3 only

G   1, 2 and 3

26   The reflex arc (from stimulus to reflex) includes the steps indicated in the flowchart below.

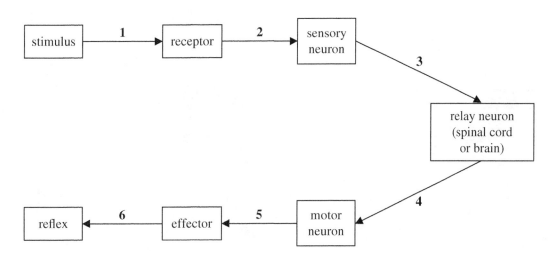

Transmitter chemicals play a role in conveying an impulse at which stages of the reflex arc?

A   2 and 3

B   3 and 4

C   4 and 5

D   2, 3 and 4

E   3, 4 and 5

F   1, 2, 5 and 6

G   All

27   The term *muzzle energy* refers to the kinetic energy of a bullet as it exits the muzzle of a gun, rifle or other firearm. Muzzle energy is carefully measured by firearms manufacturers, and it is a key selling point that might give one gun an advantage over a similar gun with a lower muzzle energy.

If a .357 Magnum pistol has muzzle energy of 750 joules and fires a bullet with an initial velocity of 360 m/s, what is the mass of a bullet fired by the .357 Magnum?

A   11.6 g

B   12.8 g

C   15.4 g

D   20.8 g

E   21.6 g

BMAT SECTION 3: WRITING TASK (30 MINUTES)

Section 3 contains a choice of three tasks. You have 30 minutes in which to answer **one**. You can take notes and make an outline in the space provided in the test booklet, but your answer must be written within the space provided on the answer sheet.

There is no correct answer to any of the questions posed. The writing task provides you with an opportunity to demonstrate your ability to:

- organise and develop your thoughts, and
- produce clear and concise written communication

Be sure to take time to organise your ideas and develop an outline. You may not use a dictionary but you may include a drawing or diagram.

Remember that you have only 30 minutes to select your task, organise your thoughts, and complete your essay.

Answer <u>one</u> of the following questions.

1   **Patients with the greatest chance of survival should be treated with the highest priority.**

Explain what this statement means. What other criteria should be used to determine the order in which patients are treated? How would you, as a doctor or veterinarian, weigh a patient's chance of survival against these other criteria?

2   **The doctor should be opaque to his patients and, like a mirror, should show them nothing but what is shown to him.**

(Sigmund Freud)

What does it mean for a doctor to be 'opaque' and 'like a mirror' to his or her patients? When might doctors find it difficult to show nothing of themselves? Is it ever acceptable for a doctor to be more than 'a mirror' to patients?

3   **Be less curious about people and more curious about ideas.**

(Marie Curie)

Could this be helpful advice for doctors? Argue to the contrary. To what extent must doctors balance their interest in ideas with their engagement with other people?

BMAT TEST 6 – ANSWER KEY

SECTION 1	
Question	Answer
1	D
2	C
3	E
4	B
5	A
6	A
7	D
8	C
9	E
10	B
11	D
12	E
13	G
14	E
15	C
16	B
17	A
18	B
19	B
20	A
21	C
22	E
23	F
24	E
25	C
26	D
27	E
28	B
29	C
30	C
31	D
32	B
33	C
34	D
35	A

SECTION 2	
Question	Answer
1	B
2	C
3	B
4	D
5	A
6	C
7	B
8	E
9	F
10	H
11	E
12	D
13	A
14	B
15	D
16	A
17	C
18	C
19	B
20	B
21	F
22	C
23	H
24	D
25	E
26	B
27	A

K

BMAT TEST 6 – SCORING TABLES

1. Count up your number of correct answers in each section. Each question is worth one mark.
2. Write the total number of marks correct in each section on the lines below.
3. Find your approximate score for each section in the table below.

	NUMBER CORRECT	APPROXIMATE BMAT SCORE
Section 1	_____	_____
Section 2	_____	_____

SECTION 1	
Number Correct	BMAT Score
0	1.0
1	1.0
2	1.0
3	1.0
4	1.0
5	1.1
6	1.5
7	1.9
8	2.2
9	2.5
10	2.8
11	3.1
12	3.4
13	3.6
14	3.9
15	4.1
16	4.4
17	4.6
18	4.9
19	5.1
20	5.4
21	5.6
22	5.9
23	6.1
24	6.4
25	6.7
26	7.0
27	7.3
28	7.6
29	8.0
30	8.4
31	8.9
32	9.0
33	9.0
34	9.0
35	9.0

SECTION 2	
Number Correct	BMAT Score
0	1.0
1	1.0
2	1.0
3	1.3
4	1.8
5	2.2
6	2.6
7	2.9
8	3.2
9	3.5
10	3.7
11	4.0
12	4.2
13	4.5
14	4.7
15	4.9
16	5.2
17	5.4
18	5.6
19	5.9
20	6.2
21	6.5
22	6.8
23	7.2
24	7.7
25	8.3
26	9.0
27	9.0

N.B. These scores are for approximation purposes only. The scoring tables used for the BMAT vary slightly year to year, depending on student performance and the norming of the questions in each version of the test paper. To err on the side of caution, these scoring tables are among the toughest ever used on the BMAT. In most cases, a similar performance on the BMAT would result in a slightly higher score.